Standardization of Quality of Life Core Outcomes in Stem Cell Clinical Trials

Dori Naerbo

DISSERTATION.COM

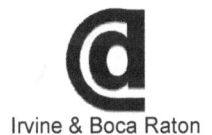

Irvine & Boca Raton

Standardization of Quality of Life Core Outcomes in Stem Cell Clinical Trials

Dissertation.com
Irvine, California • Boca Raton, Florida • USA
2018

ISBN: 978-1-61233-466-0 (pbk.)
ISBN: 978-1-61233-467-7 (ebk.)

ABSTRACT

Standardization of Quality of Life Core Outcomes in Stem Cell Clinical Trials

By Dori Naerbo, Ph.D.

Background: Establishing standardized Quality of Life (QOL) core outcomes in stem cell clinical trials is important to ensure (1) researchers and clinicians can make informed decisions, and (2) clinical trials use and consistently measure the same units (Clarke, 2007; Thornley & Adams, 1998). This study reviews the most common QOL methodologies, timing/frequency of the measurement, and outcomes in cardiovascular stem cell clinical trials.

Methods: To identify instruments, the study reviewed MEDLINE, Scopus, and US Clinical Trials Register through September 2010, and randomized BMSC controlled trials of clinical trials from 2000-2011. The trials all used the terms (bone marrow stem cell AND quality of life OR heart OR cardiac) AND cardiac AND quality of life OR QOL. The study included a Likert scale web-based questionnaire comprised of eight questions designed to assess QOL patient satisfaction post cardiovascular stem cell treatment.

Results: Of the instruments identified, the study found that bone marrow stem cell (BMSC) clinical trials used 35 different types of methodologies, whereas cardiovascular BMSC employed more consistent methodologies. Timing, frequency, and baseline were consistently measured in BMSC clinical trials, whereas cardiovascular BMSC lacked baseline consistency and were measured primarily after treatment. Cardiovascular BMSC outcomes were consistent, whereas BMSC clinical trials had multiple outcomes.

The mean participant age was 56.25 years with a minimum age of 46 years and a maximum age of 61 years. Participants generally were educated with a minimum education level of an Associate degree and a maximum degree of Doctorate. The patient satisfaction survey revealed that participants preferred yes/no questions and surveys that required less than 15 minutes to complete, received via email, easy to understand, not too personal, relevant to feelings, containing a baseline measure, and medical-condition specific.

Conclusion: QOL outcomes are rarely assessed in BMSC cardiovascular trials. Treatments are performed all over the world, and no one knows whether these treatments actually are effective. Both standardized measurements and additional studies are needed.

Word Count Abstract: 317
Word Count Thesis Body: 9888

TABLE OF CONTENTS

LIST OF TABLES

LIST OF FIGURES

ACKNOWLEDGMENTS

The researcher especially appreciates Michael Guirguis, Dissertation Advisor, for his assistance during entire process of this dissertation. In addition, special thanks to Professor Jill Wiseberg, whose insights and ideas during the dissertation class and throughout the entire process were greatly appreciated. Thanks, also, to everyone who contributed valuable input to this project.

ABBREVIATIONS

ADL   Activities of Daily Life

AHA   American Heart Association

AMI   Acute Myocardial Infarction

BMSC   Bone Marrow Stem Cell

CCS   Canadian Cardiovascular Society Angina Scale

CDC   Center for Disease Control

COMET   Core Outcome Measures in Effectiveness Trials

IP   Intellectual Property

MLHF   Minnesota Living with Heart Failure

NGT   Nominal Group Technique

NYHA   New York Heart Association

OMERACT   Outcome Measures in Rheumatology

QOL   Quality of Life

SF-36   Short Form-36

CHAPTER 1: INTRODUCTION

Background

Establishing standardized Quality of Life (QOL) core outcomes in stem cell clinical trials is important to ensure that (1) researchers and clinicians can make informed decisions and (2) clinical trials are using the same units and measuring those units in the same way (Clarke, 2007; Thornley & Adams, 1998). Standardization of outcomes is also important according to COMET (Core Outcome Measures in Effectiveness Trials) because such standardization makes "it easier to compare, contrast, and synthesize" clinical trial outcomes, while reducing bias and incongruity (University of Liverpool, 2010). However, before core outcomes in stem cell clinical trials can be established, it is necessary to describe and evaluate the QOL core outcomes currently in use. To date, some research has been conducted in the area of bone marrow stem cell (BMSC) clinical trials as shown in Tables 1 and 2. However, there remains a dearth of standardized QOL core outcome measurements in the area of cardiovascular clinical trials.

Bone Marrow Stem Cells

The history of BMSC transplants dates back to 1939 when Osgood, Riddle, and Mathews (1939) unsuccessfully transfused BMSC to a patient with aplastic anemia. In 1940, a patient purportedly recovered from aplastic anemia after Morrison and Samwick (1940) injected BMSC from several compatible donors. Mathé, a stem cell pioneer, performed the first BMSC transplants on six physicists exposed to radiation from a nuclear site accident in Yugoslavia in 1959 (Martin, 2010). Four years later, Mathé proclaimed BMSC transplantation as a cure for leukemia, and today BMSC transplantation is used as a treatment modality in certain types of cancers. Nearly 50

1

years later, Strauer et al. (2002) published one of the first stem cell cardiovascular studies. Their research demonstrated that BMSC was safe and effective for intracoronary transplantation and could be associated with myocardial regeneration and neovascularization (Strauer et al. 2002).

Currently, organ transplant demand far surpasses supply with a growing number of heart failure cases that require transplantation. From 1995 to 2011, there were 250,000 candidates age 50-64 years ("baby boomers") awaiting transplantation according to Organ Procurement and Transplant Network (2011). The United Network for Organ Sharing (2011) reported that currently there are 111,562 wait list candidates. As of March 2011, only 6,709 received organ transplants from 3,346 donors. In 2008, the American Heart Association (AHA) (2011a) reported 2,163 heart transplants, which is a decrease from the previous year of 2,210 cases in 2007. Such cases underscore the demands for innovative cardiovascular disease BMSC treatments. Today, approximately 9,500 BMSC transplants are performed annually at more than 200 international treatment centers, and the longest post-transplant survival period is 20 years (Thomas 1990).

Bone Marrow Stem Cells to Treat Cardiovascular Disease

BMSC treatment offers new hope as an alternative therapy to restore cardiac structure and vascularity in patients with non-ischemic or ischemic heart failure (Silva et al. 2004). Cardiac stem cell therapy may regenerate the myocardium by creating new heart muscle (cardiomyogenesis) or creating new pathways or vessels (angiogenesis). Of the 14 major clinical trials cited by Wei et al. (2009), the results remain inconclusive due to several factors (i.e., delivery technique, optimal dosage, best cell types, and low transdifferentiation). Additionally, none of these studies included any QOL assessments.

Quality of Life

The World Health Organization (1948a) recognized: "Health is a state of complete physical, mental, and social well-being—not merely the absence of disease, or infirmity." According to Testa and Simonso (1996), in 1973, a MEDLINE database search on "quality of life" listed only five articles; during "subsequent five-year periods, there were 195, 273, 490, and 1252 such articles." Twenty years ago, clinicians were skeptical of QOL measures, which were considered subjective and soft (Shipper, 1983):

> The scientists may use rating scales and visual analogue scales to measure pain (not the pain as such but what patients say about their pain), and they may even invent scoring systems quantifying types of handicaps; but when they talk about measuring quality of life they have gone too far. (Wulff, 1999)

QOL has been defined as a perception about one's physical and mental health over a specific time, which is dependent on one's values, goals, expectations, standards, and concerns (CDC, 2010a; WHO, 1997b; JAMA, 2002). QOL is complex system in which extrinsic life-changing factors can affect one's physical health and psychological state. Muldoon et al. (1998) identified two operational characteristics of quality of life—"objective functioning and subjective well-being." These characteristics measure the impact of illness and treatment relative to daily life activities and satisfaction. Objective functioning measures the patient's physical well-being and functional ability, whereas subjective well-being measures emotional and social well-being (Cella, 1994).

QOL is an important component of treatment efficacy. Some patients believe that QOL is more important than length of life, as a recent study funded by the European Commission indicated. The PRIMSA group and Kings College London conducted a telephone survey of 9,344 respondents. The study addressed European respondents' preference for QOL versus quantity of life from seven countries: England, Belgium, Germany, Italy, the Netherlands, Spain, and Portugal. The survey asked respondents about their priorities when faced with a life-threatening disease with limited time to live: 71% wanted to improve QOL, whereas only 4% thought both QOL and health were equally important (BMJ Blogs, 2011a; King College London, 2011).

Historically, empirical evidence was used to determine survival; however, according to Nicolau (cited in Shipper, 1983), "quality of life is a critical factor in determining survival." Patients want to know the benefits of the treatment regardless of its scientific value. Alternatively, some patients may opt to decline treatment due to the poor QOL caused by the treatment itself.

Patient satisfaction has a direct impact on QOL, and research has confirmed that patients with better QOL live longer (Fox Chase Cancer Center, 2007). Stressors, disease impact, and treatment efficacy may negatively affect QOL outcomes. Alternatively, optimism and social support may positively affect QOL outcomes; such an effect is known as the response shift model wherein patients' internal standards, values, treatment, or a change in health status occur (Ring et al., 2005; Beeken, Eiser, & Dalley, 2010).

QOL measurement in evidence-based medicine supports decision-making, resource allocation, healthcare policy, prognostic indication, and determining interventions (Donald, 2003). Such measurement is essential to determine whether treatment is efficacious or detrimental to a patient's QOL. QOL can be measured through validated questionnaires or semi-structured interviews to evaluate patients physical, functional, social, and emotional well-being. According to PROMIS (2011), at least 106 generic instruments have been used to assess an

4

expansive collection of health domains specific to an array of health conditions and diseases. In contrast, PROMIS (2011) indicated that there are only 35 cardiovascular disease disease-specific instruments.

Core Outcomes

Minimum standards are established by core outcome sets, which are assessed and documented in all health related clinical trials (University of Liverpool, 2010). Developing core outcomes in clinical trials is important for three reasons. First, core outcomes produce homogenous trials for a methodological review, whereas the analysis of heterogeneous trials may produce inconsistent results. Second, core outcomes prioritize points-of-view important to patients and clinicians, whereas non-core outcomes-based research may focus on outcomes most significant to the researcher's viewpoint. Third, core outcomes may eliminate bias by reporting specific results that are both positive and negative, whereas many trials only report positive results (Sinha, Smyth, & Williamson 2011).

Core outcomes development requires a combined consensus from authoritative specialists and patient groups. Sinha, Smyth, and Williamson (2011) discussed the dearth of guidance in core outcome development. However, the Delphi technique, which can help minimize conformity through peer pressure and dominant individuals (Dalkey, 1968), also can be used to develop core outcomes, according to Outcome Measures in Rheumatology (OMERACT) collaborators (Sinha, Smyth, & Williamson, 2011).

Additional informal and formal consensus techniques include Nominal Group Technique (NGT) and the National Institute of Health Consensus Development Conference (Murphy et al. 1998). Upon reaching consensus, the next step is to identify potential instruments to measure core outcome sets, which are reviewed for feasibility, validity, and responsiveness (Sinha, Smyth, & Williamson, 2011). One initiative that provides reporting standards guidance and the development of core outcome sets for use in therapeutic clinical practices is known as Core Outcome Measures for Effectiveness Trials (COMET).

COMET Initiative

The COMET Initiative promotes the establishment and utilization of core outcomes through the collaboration of scientific investigators and institutions (BMJ Blogs, 2010b). COMET specifically focuses on certain variables and how they are measured in response to the effects of illnesses on patients. To date, the COMET Initiative has developed core outcome sets in over 40 therapeutic areas such as cancer, rheumatology, chronic pain, and maternity care (University of Liverpool, 2010). The use of COMET's core outcome sets may enable a standardization that will allow clinicians to analyze whether QOL core outcomes have improved or declined from study to study. By standardizing QOL core outcomes, a comparative baseline can be provided with which to analyze treatment efficacy. If standardization is not developed, patients will continue to be recruited into stem cell clinical trials with no minimum standards for QOL core outcomes. As long as there are no standards, this problem of heterogeneous clinical trials will persist.

Purpose of the Study

This study addressed the research question: *What are the QOL core outcomes currently being measured in stem cell clinical trials?* The aim of this study was to describe and evaluate the quality of life core outcomes currently being measured in US and European stem cell clinical trials.

The study's objectives were to:

1. Describe the timing/frequency intervals, and methodology of QOL core outcomes being measured in bone marrow stem cell clinical trials.

2. Describe the timing/frequency intervals, and methodology of QOL core outcomes being measured in cardiovascular stem cell clinical trials.

3. Compare and contrast QOL core outcomes measured in both groups (bone marrow and cardiovascular stem cell clinical trials).

4. Assess patient satisfaction with the QOL outcomes that currently are measured in cardiovascular stem cell clinical trials.

5. Explore possible standardization of QOL core outcomes in cardiovascular stem cell clinical.

Summary

The impact of the COMET Initiative may change the way clinical trials are conducted; in other words, investigators may be able to evaluate homogeneous stem cell clinical trials with a consistent baseline. The need for research on QOL core outcomes is clear. When clinical trials lack standardized QOL core outcomes, this omission may undermine the clinical trials' efficacy, whereas research results on QOL core outcomes may influence how clinical studies are developed and used in the future. Furthermore, using the COMET Initiative as a guide, this study will evaluate the potential for using standardized core outcomes in cardiovascular BMSC clinical trials. Effectively standardized QOL core outcomes in stem cell clinical trials may produce significant treatment benefits to millions of aging people in a currently overburdened health care system.

CHAPTER 2: LITERATURE REVIEW

Heart failure is on the rise due to the increasing age of the United States' population. Additionally, the Center for Disease Control (CDC) estimated that it would "cost the United States $316.4 billion (health care services, medications, and lost productivity) in 2010" (CDC, 2010b). Similarly, in Europe, cardiovascular disease is the most deadly disease among both sexes and causes as many as half of all deaths annually (around 2 million). According to the European Heart Network (2009), cardiovascular disease costs approximately €192 billion annually. Accordingly, heart failure treatments have become increasingly important due to the high number of cases (Perin et al. 2003a) and the economic burden of those cases (Bundkirchen & Schwinger, 2004). Of the 2,426,264 deaths reported in the United States in 2006; 631,636 died of heart disease, which accounted for 26% of deaths (Heron et al., 2009; CDC, 2010b). According to Perin et al. (2003a), "no-option" heart failure patients are subjected to aggressive therapeutic interventions with "a potential yearly mortality rate as high as 50%, and for these patients, therapeutic options remain limited." Current studies suggest that BMSC treatments may offer a cost effective alternative treatment to heart failure patients.

QOL in Bone Marrow Stem Cell Research Trials

The 1990 National Cancer Institute clinical trial and QOL expert workshop addressed QOL end-point implementation (Nayfield et al. 1992). The workshop concluded that the selection of QOL core instruments should be based on the following criteria: (1) general and disease specific evaluation and (2) reliable, valid, and psychometric evaluation. The group also recommended specific timing intervals for follow-up: (1) baseline (prior to randomization), (2) pre-treatment, (3) during treatment, (4) completion or discontinuation of study, and (5) completion of study (Nayfield et al. 1992). Table 1 shows that the majority of the trials conducted between 1991–1993 did not include the 1990 workshop group recommendation, as discussed above.

Table 1 adapted from Cancer BMSC Trials (Andrykowski et al., 1995; Hjermstad & Kaasa, 1995)

	Outcomes Measure Assessment	
Author's Name	**Follow up (months)**	**QOL Instrument**
Achard & Zittoun (1992)	Before BMT, day 1,11, and 2 1 post-treatment	Modified EORTC-QLQ C30, HAD
Aeschelmann et al.(1992)	7-96 mo post-BMT	Interview, modified CJDM
Altmaier et al. (1991)	25-41 mo post-BMT	Phone interview on health, functioning
Andrykowski et al. (1989)	3-52 mo post-BMT	POMS, FLIC
Andrykowski et al. (1989)	3 times post-BMT	POMS, FLIC, SIP
Andrykowski et al. (1990)	12-96 mo post-BMT	POMS, PAIS, SIP
Adrykowski et al. (1990)	Minimum 1 year post-BMT	POMS, FLIC, SIP, PAIS
Baker et al. (1991)	6-149 mo post-BMT	Role checklist, SLDS, CSAL, POMS, BPNAS
Baruch et al. (1991)	Minimum 6 mo post-BMT	HAD, questionnaire on health, sexual function
Belec (1992)	12-38 mo post-BMT	Interview, QLI-Cancer, checklist
Chao et al. (1992)	1 year follow-up, every 3 mo, from day + 90	Phone interview
Claisse et al. (1992)	BMT performed from 1984-1989	Questionnaire with 30 selected items
Collins et al. (1989)	Days 3,7, 12 and 19 of isolation	Semi-structured interviews

Colon et al. (1991)	Review ratings of charts prior to BMT	Psychiatric history, obtained DSM III, support
Curbow et al. (1993)	6-149 mo post-BMT	Role checklist, SLDS , CSAL, POMS, BPNAS
Cust et al. (1989)	Minimum 6 mo post- BMT	Interview, designed questionnaire
Decker et al. (1989)	One week pre-BMT, 1,6.5, 12 mo post-BMT	Exercise testing, BDI
Dermatis & Lesko (1991)	Within 48 hours after admission	Questionnaire, BSI, Ways of coping list
Ersek	Pre-BMT, days 9-12, and 25-28 post-BMT	In-depth qualitative interviews
Ferrell et al. (1991)	Minimum 100 days post-BMT	BMT-QQLS as an in depth interview
Ferro et al. (1992)	Minimum 6 mo post-BMT	Interview on psychosocial functioning
Futterman et al. (1991)	Review ratings of pre-BMT charts	Psychiatric history, social support, coping
Gaston-Johansson et al. (1992)	2 days pre-BMT, 5, 10, and 20 days post-BMT	PoM, STAI, BDI, MHLC, CSQ
Grant et al. (1992)	Minimum 100 days post-BMT	QOL-BMT questionnaire
Hengeveld et al. (1988)	12-60 mo post-BMT	Interview, BDI, SCL-90
Jenkins et al. (1991)	After discharge from BMT unit	Interview, HAD, PAIS,EPQ, CIDL
Kennedy et al. (1990)	13-62 mo post-BMT (median 30)	Phone interview, semi structured
King (1988)	At time of admission and discharge	NSSQ, BDI
Larson et al. (1993)	Day 1 post-BMT, days 7-10,20-23,3O-34	SDS, POMS
Lesko et al. (1992)	Minimum 5 years from end of treatment	BSI, MHI, IES, SAS,ABCL, DSFI, cohesion
Magid et al.(1988)	Baseline pre-BMT, 1 mo post-discharge	POMS, FLIC
Mashberg (1989)	Minimum 1 year post-BMT	BSI, DAQ, IES, PAIS,DSFI
McElwain et al. (1989)	6 mo-3 years	Infection rates, pain
Mumma et al. (1992)	Minimum 1 year post-BMT (mean 47 and 64)	Interview, BSI, POMS, DAQ, IES, PAIS, DSFI

Peters et al. (1993)	Minimum 1 year post-BMT (median 2 years)	Phone interviews, FLIC, SDS
Rodrigue et al.(1993)	Pre-BMT (mean 23 days)	BDI, STAI, STAXI,MCMQ, MMPI
Schmidt et al. (1989)	Every 3 mo, 3-140 mo (median 3.6 years)	Specifically designed questionnaire
Schmidt et al. (1993)	Minimum 12 mo post-BMT	Phone or personal interviews
Smith et al. (1984)	Pre-or post-BMT, most in the peritranspl. period	Personal interview, SRE data
Steeves (1992)	Pre-BMT to day 100	Hermeneutic methods, observation, interaction
Syrjala et al. (1990)	Pre-BMT and 1 year post-BMT	SIP, BDI, BES, coping style
Syrjala et al. (1993)	Pre-BMT, 90 days and 1 year post-BMT	SIP, BSI, BDI, family cohesion, coping style
Vose et al. (1991)	13-62 mo post-BMT	Phone interview on appearance, adjustment
Winer et al. (1992)	Min. 1 year post- BMT	FLIC, SDS, PAIS, phone interview
Wingard et al. (1992)	6-149 mo post-BMT (median 47)	MOS, SLDS, CSAL
Wingard et al. (1991)	6-149 mo post-BMT	Mailed survey, health perception scale
Wolcott et al. (1986)	Min 1 year post-BMT	SAS, POMS, Simmons
Zabora et al. (1990)	Pre BMT, 6-48 mo post BMT	SI, ICC, SLDS

Table 1 adapted from (Andrykowski et al., 1995; Hjermstad and Kaasa 1995) Cancer BMSC Trials

Furthermore, Hjermstad and Kaasa (1995) reviewed 57 BMSC trials showing that only 11 incorporated a baseline assessment of QOL. Andrykowski et al. (1995) conducted one of the largest multicenter QOL BMSC trials of its time and used instruments specially designed for assessing post-BMSC QOL. However, one of the study's limitations was that QOL assessments were not validated for BMSC patients. It seems curious that such a large study would use non-validated instruments and therefore would be subject to ambiguous interpretation.

QOL assessment is fundamentally important throughout the entire life cycle of the BMSC process. Without QOL assessment, patients cannot give true informed consent, nor can they be fully aware of the full continuum of treatment outcomes. Additionally, QOL assessments augment the clinical decision-making process for the clinician and the patient (Hjermstad & Kaasa, 1995). Moreover, QOL assessments are the most consistent prognostic factors for post-transplant psychosocial problems. Consequently, pre-transplant QOL assessments identify these issues and enable clinicians to initiate intervention programs (Hjermstad & Kaasa, 1995).

However, it is not clear why the guidelines of the 1990 workshop were not fully realized or implemented in various studies. Clinical trials without QOL assessments create disparity due to ambiguous results. This inconsistency renders clinicians and patients unable to make informed decisions, as the full continuum of treatment options is not available for analysis.

QOL in Bone Marrow Stem Cell Cardiovascular Research Trials

Treating cardiovascular disease with BMSC is a novel approach that began to emerge in 2002. Perin et al. (2011b) conducted a study, which included QOL for cardiovascular BMSC. Two questionnaires were administered: (1) general Short Form-36 (SF-36) and (2) disease specific Minnesota Living with Heart Failure (MLHF). Findings included significant improvement when compared to baseline, whereas, patients in the control group showed no marked improvement over baseline (Perin et al. 2011b). This is a significant study because they include baseline measure as compared to prior studies. BMSC treatment potentially can be cost effective as noted by Mathur and Martin (2004); however; one problem is there is no intellectual property (IP) associated with autologous BMSC (Hughes, 2004). Large-scale trials would be prohibitive due to lack of funding, which is why cellular processing methods, culture medium, delivery techniques, and catheter types can vary greatly in each trial (Hughes, 2004). For this reason, many off shore clinics have emerged to take advantage of the lack of IP. The only way to educate desperate participants is to have standards.

Wei et al. (2009) cited several major clinical studies, which used BMSC in treating acute myocardial infarction (AMI). However, several interesting factors (i.e., delivery technique, optimal dosage, best cell types, and low transdifferentiation) further illustrate the inconsistency in clinical trial methodology. Interestingly, none of the aforementioned studies cited by Wei et al. (2009) included any QOL assessments.

Several 2002-2011 cardiovascular BMSC clinical studies revealed problems with QOL, such as inconsistent QOL assessment and irregularities in timing/frequency of follow-up with patients. Furthermore, the studies had other flaws, such as treatment timing, delivery techniques, optimal dosage, and the best cell types. For example, the best time to treat acute myocardial infarct (AMI) with BMSC is between 5-14 days. This timing is based upon two factors: (1) five days after an AMI the inflammation process is the most intense and for this reason, BMSC is not recommended; and (2) scar tissue formation occurs 14 days post AMI (Yousef et al. 2009). Table 2 shows that AMI studies tend to administer the stem cells at different times. Time of administration may affect treatment efficacy and QOL; however, these outcomes cannot be determined because they are not measured.

Table 2: AMI Transplant Days in BMSC Trials

Study Name	Study Type	Transplant (Days)
ASTAMI (Norway) Lunde et al. 2005	AMI	5-9 d
BALANCE (Germany) Yousef et al. (2009)	AMI	7 ± 2 d
BOOST (Germany) Wollert et al. 2004	AMI	5d
BONAMI (France) Roncalli et al. 2010	AMI	7–10 d
REPAIR-AMI (Germany) Schächinger et al. 2006	AMI	3 – 7 d
Strauer et al. 2002 (Germany)	AMI	5-9 d
TOPCARE-AMI (Germany) Assmus et al. 2002	AMI	4.3±1.5 d

Delivery techniques varied from study to study. For example, Lunde et al. (2005) and Yousef et al. (2009) used angioplasty balloon catheter to deliver BMSC; however, Yousef et al. (2009) used twice the number of stem cells and a different delivery technique. One could argue plausibly that some patients experienced the same benefits from angioplasty with or without BMSC. Perhaps some patients obtained benefit solely from angioplasty, which restores blood flow, as opposed to receiving benefits strictly from BMSC treatments. BMSC trials draw disparate amounts of bone marrow, and determination of optimal dosage is not yet established (Lunde et al., 2005; Schächinger et al., 2006; Perin et al., 2003a; Roncalli et al., 2010; Patel et al., 2005; and

Yousef et al., 2009). The diversity in trial results may be attributed to the different amounts of aspirated cells. Nevertheless, this area requires further investigation.

The majority of BMSC heart failure studies use some form of assessment like QOL or functional class, whereas AMI studies typically do not. The heterogeneity of the trials combined with the dearth of longitudinal QOL studies make treatment efficacy difficult to evaluate.

Quality of Life Assessments

The standardization of QOL outcomes in stem cell clinical trials also must consider the type of instrument used to measure outcomes (Mosher, 2010; Le et al., 2010; and Slovacek, 2007). A study of 2,000 controlled trials in schizophrenia over a 50-year period concluded that all clinical research benefits from standardization (Thornlay & Adams, 1998). The researchers identified the use of 600 different rating scales, which could result in a lack of statistical power. Their findings further illustrated the need for creating a disease or condition-specific core set of outcomes for use in clinical trials. For example, Nayfield et al. (1992) discussed a core set of QOL outcome recommendations that divided cancer into four groups:

1. Generic instruments: general medical conditions (i.e., Medical Outcomes Study [MOS] Short Form [SF])

2. Generic instruments (i.e., cancer; see Cancer Rehabilitation Evaluation System [CARES])

3. Disease/site-specific instruments (i.e., EORTC Modules for Disease Sites)

4. Dimension-specific instruments (i.e., Psychosocial Adjustment to Illness Scale-Self-Report version [PAIS-SR])

Heterogeneous BMSC clinical trials currently use disparate types of QOL assessments (Figure 1) and inconsistent timing/frequency follow-up intervals, which is problematic when evaluating whether QOL has improved or declined from study to study. For example, the study by Willerson et al. (2010) notably failed to assess patient QOL prior to transplant in terms of whether patients improved, deteriorated, or demonstrated no measureable changes. This is an important issue because patients can experience significant results at three and six months and the study can be touted as a success. However, without baseline and long-term follow-up QOL assessments, placebo effects cannot be taken into consideration.

Assessment: Short Form-36 (SF-36)

Early BMSC trials lacked QOL core outcomes, but they showed post-transplant improvement and the need for further QOL research. Lunde et al. (2005) was the first BMSC clinical trial to include QOL assessment with SF-36; however, they failed to report any QOL results.

Assessment: The Minnesota Living with Heart Failure (MLHF)

The Minnesota Living with Heart Failure (MLHF) instrument assesses a patient's QOL based on the treatment and how it affects heart failure (University of Minnesota, 2010). Recently, QOL instruments are gaining more credibility in BMSC clinical trials as exemplified by the ongoing clinical trial IMPACT (NCT01020968) and PERFECT (NCT00950274T) trials, which assess QOL with MLHF. One study assessed QOL with SF-36 and the MLHF questionnaire in an effort to have a comprehensive examination, but it did not obtain findings from one assessment or the other (Willerson et al. 2010).

Outcomes with NYHA and CCS

The New York Heart Association (NYHA) and Canadian Cardiovascular Society (CCS)

Angina Scale functional class is determined by symptomatology. NYHA and CCS are also

synonymous with QOL and activities of daily life (ADL). Coyne & Allen (1998) made a valid

point in the evaluation of functional class: functional class ratings are subject to ambiguous

interpretation because patients can adapt their activities to avoid symptoms, when in fact, they have

not improved their functional class at all. The NYHA and CCS functional classifications were

introduced as secondary endpoints in BMSC clinical trials (Patel et al. 2005). In an effort to reduce

investigators' bias with functional classifications, investigators were not allowed access to the

clinical assessments. Several studies included NYHA and SF36; however, there is no consistency

in whether they included one, the other, or both—such lack of consistency adds to the discrepancy

in measuring outcomes.

Timing/Frequency Follow up

Cancer BMSC QOL outcomes are typically measured pre, during, and post transplant

regardless of the number of months transpiring (Packman et al. 2010). By contrast, cardiovascular

BMSC studies measure QOL outcomes post-treatment at 3, 6, and 12-month intervals (Willerson

et al. 2010). Neither framework accounts for QOL measurement timing. Furthermore, many

cancer BMSC trials include a baseline QOL assessment; conversely, most cardiovascular BMSC

studies do not. Moreover, long-term follow-up studies in cancer BMSC trials help to determine

treatment effects such as toxicity of treatment. However, cardiovascular BMSC treatment is a

newly emerging medical field, and for this reason, long-term follow-up studies are limited.

Additionally, many cancer and cardiovascular interventions are painful, uncomfortable, and stressful, which may lead to post traumatic stress disorder and depression. The full extent of the psychological stressors consequently is unknown due to inconsistent timing/frequency measures, which indicates that comparative timing/frequency analysis is problematic (Meyers et al. 1994). QOL timing/frequency follow-up measures are important because they provide invaluable information to the clinician, empower patients to have a voice, and identify underlying stressors.

Summary

The literature review shows that incorporating QOL core outcomes in clinical trials is well documented in cancer BMSC trials. Conversely, QOL core outcomes in cardiovascular BMSC trials essentially are absent from the literature. Some cardiovascular BMSC trials used inconsistent QOL assessment scales and failed to report results; nonetheless, they reported subjective functional class changes. Furthermore, incongruent timing/frequency obfuscates critical evaluations for appropriate treatment options. The inconsistency between multiple QOL rating scales, timing/frequency, and heterogeneity in BMSC clinical trials warrants further evaluation. In order to reduce the number of patients lost to follow-up, the study reported herein assessed patient satisfaction with the QOL outcomes currently measured in cardiovascular stem cell clinical trials.

CHAPTER 3: METHODOLOGY

Research Design

A quantitative research design was selected for this study. Quantitative research is characterized by confirmation, deduction, data collection, and statistical analysis (Creswell, 2003). The study was suggestive and the participation was voluntary. There were no control groups. There were no assumptions made about whether participants had preconceived opinions or attitudes. Since the researcher has extensive experience in autologous stem cells, the researcher merely observed and no attempts were made to influence participants' attitudes.

Suitability of Design

It was determined that a quantitative, descriptive research design was the most suitable based on the type of data from participants in a specific demographics of (1) previously treated participants and (2) the majority of the published clinical trials. This design allowed the researcher to evaluate relationships between groups (i.e. BMSC clinical trials and cardiovascular BMSC clinical trials). Additionally, it allowed the researcher to deduce the possibility of certain relationships based on the research and its variables.

Research Questions

1. Which timing/frequency intervals and methodology of QOL core outcomes are measured in bone marrow stem cell clinical trials?

2. Which timing/frequency intervals and methodology of QOL core outcomes are measured in cardiovascular stem cell clinical trials?

3. What is the difference in QOL core outcomes between groups (bone marrow and cardiovascular stem cell clinical trials)?

4. How is patient satisfaction with the QOL outcomes assessed as currently measured in cardiovascular stem cell clinical trials?

How can research develop possible standardization of QOL core outcomes in cardiovascular stem cell clinical trials?

Literature Review Methods

This study was a contrastive literature review of QOL outcomes in bone marrow and cardiovascular stem cell clinical trials.

Literature Review Search Strategy

The search strategy included MEDLINE, Scopus, and US Clinical Trials Register through September 2010 for English language, randomized controlled trials of BMSC clinical trials from 2000 -2011. The relevant materials search included, but was not limited to, libraries catalogues, databases, Internet, and bibliographies. Search terms included: bone marrow stem cell, bone marrow stem cell transplant, quality of life, cardiac, heart, stem cell transplantation, hematopoietic stem cell transplantation and cardiovascular stem cell transplant.

Search strategy inclusion criteria.

Literature review included: (a) studies conducted from 2000-2010 for BMSC transplants in cancer patients and (b) studies conducted from 2005- to present for BMSC cardiovascular patients.

Search strategy exclusion criteria.

The exclusion criteria included all works that are unpublished in peer-reviewed journals (i.e., conference papers, master's theses, doctoral dissertations, and unpublished working papers).

Search Parameters

Scopus search queries included: bone marrow stem cell transplant, bone marrow stem cell transplant AND quality of life, bone marrow stem cell AND quality of life, bone marrow stem cell AND heart, bone marrow stem cell AND cardiac, and bone marrow stem cell AND cardiac AND QOL.

Clinical Trial.gov search parameter included: bone marrow stem cells and bone marrow stem cells AND QOL.

Medline search queries included: bone marrow stem cell AND quality of life (Broad search), bone marrow stem cell AND quality of life (Narrow search), and bone marrow stem cell AND cardiac AND quality of life. The broad and narrow searches are a type of filter to expand or limit search queries (e.g., a narrow search only includes the specific search criteria).

Survey Methods

Population and Sample

Participants were sampled from the Stem Cell Pioneer Board to participate in a QOL patient satisfaction survey. All participants in the population received BMSC treatment. Given time constraints and since participants were immediately available, it was decided that convenience sampling would be used (Neuman, 2003). It should be noted that random sampling would have made the study more reproducible, however.

Patient Survey Source Selection

The Stem Cell Pioneers forum was selected for the patient satisfaction survey. The anticipated number of participants was 15-30. The Stem Cell Pioneer board sample included primarily USA based participants located in urban areas. The population group was diverse. Patients were recruited voluntarily by two methods:

1. A recruitment message for study volunteers was posted on the Stem Cell Pioneers Board. The message explained that qualified participants (patients previously treated with autologous stem cells) were being sought for a QOL Study investigating how treated outcomes are measured. Those interested were asked to contact the student investigator by email. The potential participants were then screened for eligibility during a brief telephone call.

2. A random sampling of treated patients from a private autologous stem cell company were drawn from a list, contacted by email, and invited to participate in the study. These participants needed to meet the eligibility requirements outlined below.

Eligibility requirements included that participants needed to be 18-75 years of age, post-autologous stem cell treatment patients, and were administered QOL questionnaires. Following the administration of the questionnaire, all data were coded, verified, and analyzed as percentages.

Patient QOL Survey

The study included a Likert scale web-based questionnaire comprised of eight questions designed to assess QOL patient satisfaction that have received cardiovascular stem cell treatments. All questions except for question 2 and 8 were scaled using a 5-point scaling strategy where options ranged from Strongly Disagree to Strongly Agree. Question 2 asked participants the type of survey they completed, while question 8 asked participants about gender, age, educational degree, and address. Survey Money was used to develop and host the free online questionnaire.

Data Analysis

The Statistical Package for the Social Sciences (SPSS) software program, Student Version 17.0 was used to analyze the data.

Ethical Considerations

Ethical concerns for this study included (1) voluntary participation, (2) truthful and sincere data, and (3) participants to follow instructions when answering the patient satisfaction QOL survey, which was used for data compilation.

Informed Consent. All participants needed to read and accept an online informed consent form before proceeding with the patient satisfaction QOL survey.

Voluntary Participation. Participation was voluntarily and participants had the right to discontinue involvement at any time during the survey.

Confidentiality. No information that could possibly identify the participant was disclosed or will be published, and all information is confidential. Results are presented as summative, median data.

Risks and Benefits. There were no risks for being in the study. The study may benefit research and may improve the understanding of QOL and its importance in cardiovascular BMSC trials.

Summary

Participant selections were based upon (1) prior treatment with stem cells and (2) having previously completed a QOL questionnaire. Participant selection was voluntary throughout the entire process. The researcher had prior experience with stem cell participants, but acted only has an observer. Data gathering was sparse for QOL cardiovascular stem cell trials in peer reviewed literature. To account for the lack of data, trial boards (i.e., clinical trials.gov) were used to supplement the literature gap. The rational for data analysis was dependent upon the number of responses in the patient satisfaction survey.

CHAPTER 4: RESULTS

BMSC cardiovascular clinical trials research lacks standardized QOL core outcome measurements. Accordingly, this study investigated the following research questions to ameliorate this research gap:

1. Which timing/frequency intervals and methodology of QOL core outcomes are measured in bone marrow stem cell clinical trials?

2. Which timing/frequency intervals and methodology of QOL core outcomes are measured in cardiovascular stem cell clinical trials?

3. What is the difference in QOL core outcomes between groups (bone marrow and cardiovascular stem cell clinical trials)?

4. How is patient satisfaction with the QOL outcomes assessed as currently measured in cardiovascular stem cell clinical trials?

5. How can research develop possible standardization of QOL core outcomes in cardiovascular stem cell clinical trials?

Selection Results

Ongoing BMSC Trials Selection Results

There were 87 ongoing BMSC clinical trials identified at clinicaltrials.gov and 31 studies were identified that included the search parameters bone marrow stem cells AND QOL. Terminated; suspended studies or those that did not meet the criteria were not included. Next, the data were organized into the appropriate categories: Instruments/Methodology, Timing/Frequency and Outcomes. Of the 31 trials, the study investigated 17 ongoing BMSC clinical trials and 14 ongoing cardiovascular BMSC trials.

Literature Review Selection Results

There were 14 completed studies identified from the literature review that were selected. The search parameters used were too broad, which produced studies that were not applicable. Therefore, cardiovascular studies were located by general Internet searches. Once a suitable study that met the criteria was located, it was cross-referenced into Scopus, Medline, and clinicaltrials.gov in order to narrow the search parameter terms for suitable studies. Next, the study references were reviewed to find links to similar studies.

BMSC Ongoing Clinical Trials Results

The timing/frequency intervals and methodology of QOL core outcomes measured in BMSC clinical studies were investigated in 17 ongoing BMSC clinical trials. Instrument/Methodology, Timing/Frequency, and Outcomes were specified as evaluative points.

Instrument

From research, 35 different types of instruments/methodology were identified as commonly used, but only 17 were directly associated with bone marrow stem cell clinical trials. These included SCL-90-R, CTXD, EORTC QLQ-C30, Short Form SF-36, Heath Assessment Questionnaire (HAQ), Harris Hip Score, Visual Analogue Scale (VAS), Oswestry disability index, WOMAC osteoarthritis Index, City of Hope, short Inflammatory Bowel Disease Questionnaire (sIBDQ), FACT, FACT-G, FACT-BMT, Brief Cope, SDS, and POMS. The most likely instrument/methodology used was the Short Form SF-36 with five of the 17 studies using this method. Three of the seventeen studies used a Visual Analogue Scale (VAS) to assess QOL while the rest of the instruments were used only once across the different studies.

Timing and Frequency

There were 13 criteria identified from research that represented different intervals used in the 17 selected studies. The intervals were divided into three logical groups including *Baseline*, *Baseline with Post Baseline*, and *Post Baseline without Baseline*. Results from the research found that one of the 17 studies used Baseline only, six used baseline with follow-up, and eleven of the 17 used QOL surveys after surgery without baseline information. Five of the six studies used baseline with multiple follow-ups while only one study used a single follow-up after baseline evaluation.

Outcomes

Twelve outcomes were identified from research including disease free survival, disease free interval, adverse events, quality of life, psychosocial behavior, physical, cognitive, neuroendocrine, GVHD, safety and efficacy, LVEF changes, and decrease in NYHA. Two of the seventeen studies assessed a combination of the first four outcomes while one of the studies measured psychosocial behavior, physical, cognitive, neuroendocrine, and GVHD. A single study measured disease free survival.

Cardiovascular BMSC Ongoing Clinical Trials Results

The timing/frequency intervals and methodology of QOL core outcomes measured in cardiovascular bone marrow stem cell clinical studies were investigated in 14 ongoing clinical trials.

Instrument

From research, 35 different types of instruments/methodology were identified as commonly used, but only six were directly associated with cardiovascular stem cell clinical trials. These included Rand 36, SF-36, Kansas City Cardiomyopathy, Minnesota Living with Heart Failure, Seattle Angina, and EQ-5D. The most frequently used instrument/methodology was the SF-36 with four of the 14 studies using this method. Three of the 14 studies used the Minnesota Living with Heart Failure to assess QOL while three of the studies used the EQ-5D. The remaining instruments were used only once across the different studies.

Timing and Frequency

There were 13 timing criteria identified from research used in the 14 selected studies. The intervals were divided into three logical groups including *Baseline, Baseline with Post Baseline,* and *Post Baseline without Baseline.* Results from the research found that none of the 14 studies used Baseline only while five used baseline with follow-up and nine of the 14 used QOL surveys after surgery without baseline information. The most common timing (two of four studies) was baseline with 6 month or 12 month follow-up. Three of the four studies that used baseline with follow-up administered multiple follow-up surveys.

Outcomes

Thirteen outcomes were identified from research including disease free survival, disease free interval, adverse events, quality of life, psychosocial behavior, physical, cognitive, neuroendocrine, GVHD, safety and efficacy, LVEF Changes, Decrease in NYHA, and Amputation. Three of the fourteen studies assessed safety and efficacy while six of the fourteen studies examined LVEF Changes. Two studies examined adverse advents and two studies examined amputation. Only one study examined decrease in NYHA.

Cardiovascular BMSC Trials Literature Review Results

The timing/frequency intervals and methodology of QOL core outcomes measured in cardiovascular stem cell clinical trials was explored by reviewing 14 completed cardiovascular stem cell clinical trials (see Table 4). Table 4 shows 14 cardiovascular BMSC trials (2002-2011) that incorporated QOL assessment, timing/frequency, and other clinical assessment scales (e.g., NYHA and Canadian Cardiovascular Society Angina Scale [CCS]). Additionally, eight ongoing cardiovascular BMSC clinical trials were investigated. Instrument/Methodology, Timing/Frequency, and Outcomes were specified as evaluative points.

Table 3 Cardiovascular BMSC Trials (2002-2011)

| | Study Name | Study Type | Transplant (Days) | Outcomes Measure Assessment | | |
				Follow up (months)	QOL Instrument	Secondary Outcomes
1	ASTAMI (Norway) Lunde et al. 2005	AMI	5-9 d	1 and 6	SF 36	
2	BALANCE (Germany) Yousef et al. 2009	AMI	7 ± 2 d		None	
3	BOOST (Germany) Wollert et al., 2004	AMI	5d		None	
4	BONAMI (France) Roncalli et al. 2010	AMI	7–10 d		None	
5	FOCUS (USA) Willerson et al. 2010	HF		3 and 6	SF-36 MLHF	NYHA, CCS
6	IMPACT (USA) ClinicalTrials.gov Identifier: NCT01020968	HF		Baseline, 3, 6 and 12	MLHF	NYHA, CCS
7	Patel et al. 2005 (USA)	HF			None	NYHA
8	Perin et al. 2003 (USA)	HF			None	NYHA, CCS
9	PERFECT (Germany) ClinicalTrials.gov Identifier: NCT00950274	MI + CABG		3 and 6	MLHF, SF36,EQ-5D	NYHA, CCS
10	REPAIR-AMI (Germany) Schächinger et al. 2006	AMI	3 – 7 d		None	NYHA
11	Strauer et al. 2002 (Germany)	AMI	5-9 d		None	
12	TOPCARE-AMI (Germany) Assmus et al. 2002	AMI	4.3±1.5 d		None	

Figure 1 represents the most common QOL assessment used in BMSC cardiovascular trials from 2002–2011 based on the studies in Table 3. Nearly 70% of these studies do not measure QOL. Of the studies that measured QOL, 25% used EQ-5D, 75% used both SF-36 and MLHF.

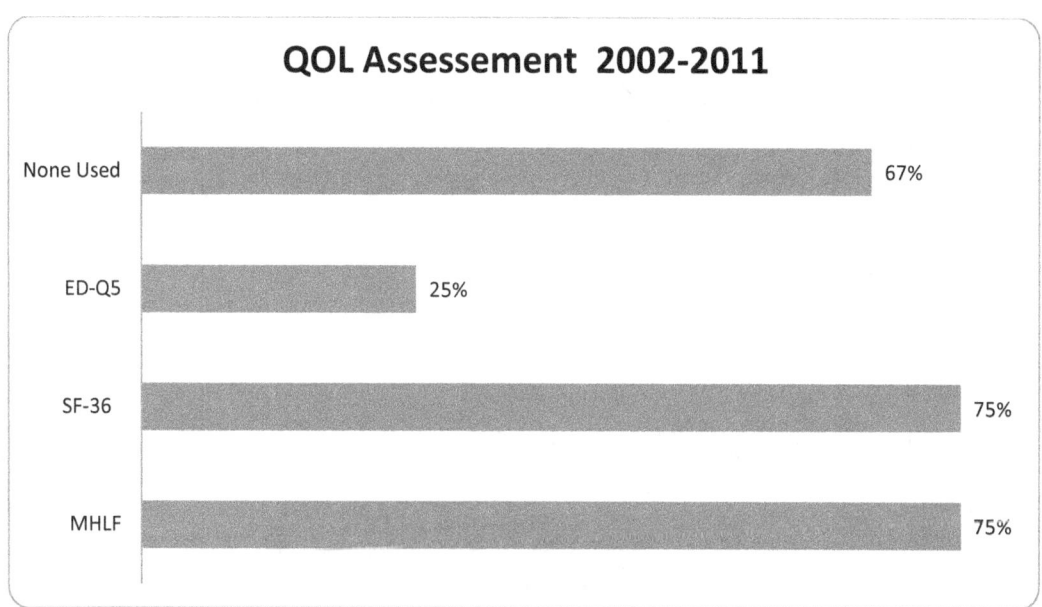

Figure 1: QOL Assessments Based on Table 3

Figure 2 represents timing/frequency of follow up used in BMSC cardiovascular trials from 2002–2011 based on the studies shown in Table 3. The majority of the studies that measured QOL limited follow up intervals to baseline, three months, six months and twelve months.

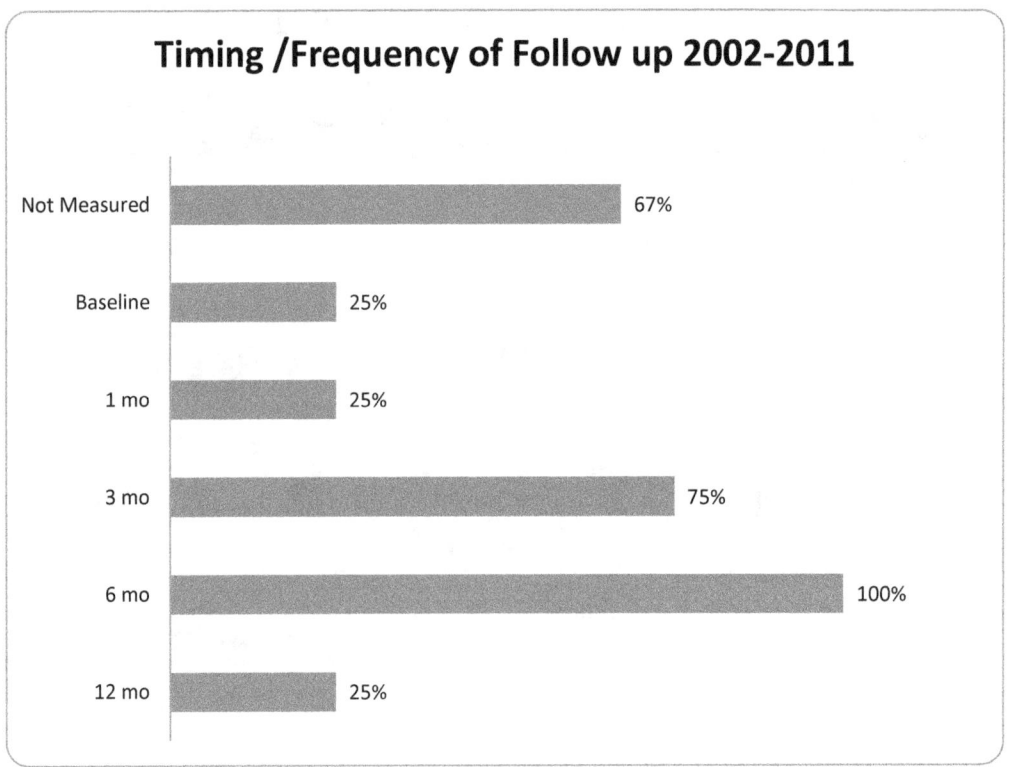

Figure 2: Timing and Frequency Based on Table 3

QOL core outcomes measured in both groups (bone marrow and cardiovascular) stem cell clinical trials were compared. Comparing core outcomes between bone marrow and cardiovascular clinical trials produced relevant findings. BMSC clinical trials outcomes measured disease free survival, disease free interval, adverse events, quality of life, psychosocial behavior, safety, and efficacy. However, cardiovascular BMSC outcomes focused on LVEF Changes and decrease in NYHA classification.

Patient QOL Survey Results

To determine whether patients were satisfied with the QOL outcomes currently measured in cardiovascular stem cell clinical trials, a questionnaire was administered. A survey containing six Likert scale questions was sent to patients that received stem cell treatment and completed a QOL survey.

Data Analysis Results

The results were presented in sequential order. The demographic section includes a profile of participants responding to the survey. Specifically, gender, age, and education level were reported using frequency statistics. This data analysis section includes descriptive statistics, means, standard deviation, and frequency where applicable.

Demographics

Ten participants opened and viewed the QOL survey; however, only four participants completed the eight-item questionnaire. Respondents included two males and two females from the USA. The mean participant age was 56.25 years with a minimum age of 46 years and a maximum age of 61 years. Participants generally were educated with a minimum education level of an Associate degree and a maximum degree of Doctorate. See Table 4 for details.

Table 4: Descriptive Demographic Information about Participants

Demographics	Count	Average
Gender		
Male	2	
Female	2	
Average Age	4	56.25
Highest Degree		
Associate	1	
Bachelor's	1	
MBA	1	
Doctorate	1	

Question 1 asked participants to make preference choices for the following: *"I thought the quality of live questionnaire was: (too personal, too complicated, too time consuming, too long,* and *hard to understand)."* Patients were instructed to answer each sub question to the best of their ability using a 5-point Likert type scale that ranged from strongly disagree to agree. Despite efforts to encourage participation, only two patients responded to survey question 1. As displayed in the table, patients did not necessarily feel that the QOL survey was *too personal*, *too long*, or *too time consuming*. No response was recorded for *too complicated* or *hard to understand*.

36

Table 3: Descriptive Percentages and Frequency Counts by Sub-question for Question 1

1. I thought the Quality of Life questionnaire was:	Strongly Disagree	Disagree	Neither	Agree	Strongly Agree	Rating Average	Response Count
Too personal	0.0% (0)	50.0% (1)	50.0% (1)	0.0% (0)	0.0% (0)	2.5	2
Too complicated	0.0% (0)	0.0% (0)	0.0% (0)	0.0% (0)	0.0% (0)	0	0
Too time consuming	0.0% (0)	0.0% (0)	100.0% (1)	0.0% (0)	0.0% (0)	3	1
Too long	0.0% (0)	0.0% (0)	100.0% (1)	0.0% (0)	0.0% (0)	3	1
Hard to understand	50.0% (1)	50.0% (1)	0.0% (0)	0.0% (0)	0.0% (0)	1.5	2

Question 2, as shown in Table 6, asked participants to make preference choices for the following: "*I prefer the Quality of Life survey to be administered by: (telephone, email, office visit, IPad,* and *web-based self-administered)*." Patients were instructed to answer each sub question to the best of their ability using a 5-point Likert type scale that ranged from strongly disagree to agree. Three patients responded survey question 2. As displayed in the table, patients preferred *email* to *telephone, office visit,* or *IPad* with three indicating *strongly agree* to *email.* No response was recorded for *telephone, office visit,* or *IPad*. One respondent strongly disagreed with web-based administration while another patient *agreed* with the method of delivery.

Table 4: Descriptive Percentages and Frequency Counts by Sub-question for Question 2

2. I prefer the Quality of Life survey to be administered by	Strongly Disagree	Disagree	Neither	Agree	Strongly Agree	Rating Average	Response Count
Telephone	0.0% (0)	0.0% (0)	0.0% (0)	0.0% (0)	0.0% (0)	0.00	0
Email	33.3% (1)	0.0% (0)	0.0% (0)	0.0% (0)	66.7% (2)	3.67	3
Office Visit	0.0% (0)	0.0% (0)	0.0% (0)	0.0% (0)	0.0% (0)	0.00	0
IPad	0.0% (0)	0.0% (0)	0.0% (0)	0.0% (0)	0.0% (0)	0.00	0
Web-based self-administered	50.0% (1)	0.0% (0)	0.0% (0)	50.0% (1)	0.0% (0)	2.50	2

Question 3 asked participants to make preference choices for the following: "*I think Quality of Life survey should be administered: (before treatment, during treatment, 1 month after,*

3 months after, 6 months after, 1 year after, and *2 years after*)." Patients were instructed to answer

each sub question to the best of their ability using a 5-point Likert type scale that ranged from

strongly disagree to strongly agree. As shown in Table 7, six of ten patients responded to survey

question 3. One of the six participants answered *agree* to before and during treatment. Four of the

six participants preferred administration after treatment while two preferred before treatment. Only

one participant strongly disagreed with administration of QOL survey three months after treatment.

Table 5: Descriptive Percentages and Frequency Counts by Sub-question for Question 3

3. I think Quality of Life survey should be administered	Strongly disagree	Disagree	Neither	Agree	Strongly agree	Rating Average	Response Count
Before treatment	0.0% (0)	0.0% (0)	0.0% (0)	50.0% (1)	50.0% (1)	4.5	2
During treatment	0.0% (0)	0.0% (0)	0.0% (0)	100.0% (1)	0.0% (0)	4	1
1 month after treatment	0.0% (0)	0.0% (0)	0.0% (0)	0.0% (0)	0.0% (0)	0	0
3 months after treatment	50.0% (1)	0.0% (0)	0.0% (0)	0.0% (0)	50.0% (1)	3	2
6 months after treatment	0.0% (0)	0.0% (0)	0.0% (0)	100.0% (1)	0.0% (0)	4	1
1 year after treatment	0.0% (0)	0.0% (0)	0.0% (0)	0.0% (0)	100.0% (1)	5	1
2 years after treatment	0.0% (0)	0.0% (0)	0.0% (0)	0.0% (0)	100.0% (1)	5	1

Question 4 asked participants to make preference choices for the following: "*I think the*

Quality of Life questions were relevant to: (my condition, my feelings, what I was expecting, and

my emotional well being)." Patients were instructed to answer each sub question to the best of their

ability using a 5-point Likert type scale that ranged from strongly disagree to strongly agree. Four

of ten patients responded to survey question 4, as shown in Table 8. Three of four participants

either *agreed* or *strongly agreed* to *my condition* while one replied *neither*. One participant *agreed*

that the QOL survey was relevant to his/her feelings. No responses were recorded for *what I was*

experiencing or *my emotional well-being.*

Table 6: Descriptive Percentages and Frequency Counts by Sub-question for Question 4

4. I think the Quality of Life questions were relevant to	Strongly disagree	Disagree	Neither	Agree	Strongly agree	Rating Average	Response Count
My condition	0.0% (0)	0.0 % (0)	25. 0% (1)	25.0 % (1)	50. 0% (2)	4.2 5	4
My feelings	0.0% (0)	0.0 % (0)	0.0 % (0)	100. 0% (1)	0.0 % (0)	4	1
What I was experiencing	0.0% (0)	0.0 % (0)	0.0 % (0)	0.0 % (0)	0.0 % (0)	0	0
My emotional well-being	0.0% (0)	0.0 % (0)	0.0 % (0)	0.0 % (0)	0.0 % (0)	0	0

Question 5 asked participants to make preference choices for the following: "*I would prefer to complete a Quality of Life questionnaire provided it took: (10 min, 15 min, 30 min, or 60 min.*" Patients were instructed to answer each sub question to the best of their ability using a 5-point Likert type scale that ranged from strongly disagree to strongly agree. As seen in Table 9, four of ten patients responded to survey question 5. Three of four participants either *agreed* or *strongly agreed* to *10 minutes* while one replied *either*. One participant strongly *agreed* that the QOL survey should take 15 minutes. No responses were recorded for *30 minutes* or *60 minutes*.

Table 7: Descriptive Percentages and Frequency Counts by Sub-question for Question 5

1. I would prefer to complete a Quality of Life questionnaire provided it took	Strongly disagree	Disagree	Neither	Agree	Strongly agree	Rating Average	Response Count
10 minutes	0.0 % (0)	0.0 % (0)	0.0 % (0)	66. 7% (2)	33. 3% (1)	4.3 3	3
15 minutes	0.0 % (0)	0.0 % (0)	0.0 % (0)	0.0 % (0)	10 0.0% (1)	5	1
30 minutes	0.0 % (0)	0.0 % (0)	0.0 % (0)	0.0 % (0)	0.0 % (0)	0	0
60 minutes	0.0 % (0)	0.0 % (0)	0.0 % (0)	0.0 % (0)	0.0 % (0)	0	0

Question 6 asked participants to make preference choices for the following: "*I prefer this format when answering questionnaires: (one answer, multiple choice, essay, or rating scale).*" Patients were instructed to answer each sub question to the best of their ability using a 5-point

Likert-type scale that ranged from strongly disagree to strongly agree. Four of ten patients

responded to survey question 6, as shown in Table 10. Two participants either *agreed* or *strongly*

agreed to *one answer questions* while one replied *strongly agree* to *essay* and one participant

strongly agreed to rating scale.

Table 8: Descriptive Percentages and Frequency Counts by Sub-question for Question 6

1. I prefer this format when answering questionnaires	Strongly disagree	Disagree	Neither	Agree	Strongly agree	Rating Average	Response Count
One answer (Yes/no)	0.0 % (0)	0.0 % (0)	0.0 % (0)	50. 0% (1)	50.0 % (1)	4.5	2
Multiple Choice (multiple answers)	0.0 % (0)	0.0 % (0)	0.0 % (0)	0.0 % (0)	0.0 % (0)	0	0
Essay /Comments	0.0 % (0)	0.0 % (0)	0.0 % (0)	0.0 % (0)	100. 0% (1)	5	1
Rating Scale (1, 2, 3, 4, 5)	0.0 % (0)	0.0 % (0)	0.0 % (0)	0.0 % (0)	100. 0% (1)	5	1

Summary

BMSC clinical trials used 35 different types of methodologies, whereas cardiovascular

BMSC employed more consistent methodologies. Timing and frequency measured baseline

consistently in BMSC clinical trials, whereas cardiovascular BMSC lacked baseline consistency

and measured primarily after treatment. Cardiovascular BMSC outcomes were consistent, whereas

BMSC clinical trials had multiple outcomes.

The patient satisfaction survey was limited but revealed that participants preferred yes/no

questions, surveys that required less than 15 minutes to complete, were received via email, were

easy to understand, were not too personal, were relevant to feelings, contained a baseline measure,

and were medical condition specific.

CHAPTER 5. DISCUSSION

The purpose of this quantitative study was to describe and evaluate the QOL core outcomes currently measured in stem cell clinical trials. QOL is an important component of treatment efficacy. Establishing standardized QOL core outcomes in stem cell clinical trials may ensure that researchers and clinicians can make informed decisions and that clinical trials use and measure the same units consistently (Clarke, 2007; Thornley & Adams, 1998). Additionally, core outcomes produce homogenous trials for systematic review, which is necessary because heterogeneous trials analysis impedes accurate synthesis. Furthermore, core outcomes prioritize points-of-view important to patients and clinicians, whereas non-core outcomes-based research may focus on outcomes most significant to the researcher's viewpoint. Finally, core outcomes may eliminate bias by reporting specific results that are both positive and negative, whereas many trials only report positive results (Sinha, Smyth, & Williamson 2011).

A review of the literature showed that incorporating QOL core outcomes in clinical trials is well documented in cancer BMSC trials. Conversely, QOL core outcomes in cardiovascular BMSC trials essentially are absent from the literature. However, some cardiovascular BMSC trials used inconsistent QOL assessment scales and failed to report results; nonetheless, they reported subjective functional class changes. Furthermore, incongruent timing/frequency obfuscates critical evaluations for appropriate treatment options.

To date BMSC cardiovascular researchers have overlooked the correlation between QOL and treatment efficacy. Research shows that extrapolation of data from peer research is not done as exemplified by different treatment times, delivery techniques, optimal dosage, and cell types used in clinical trials. Furthermore, QOL is rarely assessed in BMSC cardiovascular trials. The

41

exclusion of QOL outcome measures in several BMSC trials is a matter of pure speculation. In an attempt to determine the reason for this lack of QOL assessment, the researcher emailed Wollert et al., (2004), Patel et al., (2005), Schächinger et al., (2006), Yousef et al., (2009), and Roncalli et al., (2010); they were asked why QOL was not included in their respective studies. Out of the five study authors, only one responded: the QOL data was available but not evaluated and, therefore, excluded from the results. Investigators need irrefutable evidence to validate scientific results. It is plausible that QOL assessments were not included in some studies in order to reduce the chance of bias. However, it is important that investigators report all results and not withhold any important information. Without QOL assessment at baseline, whether treatment is effect or placebo remains unknown.

Summary of Results

An examination was conducted of timing/frequency intervals and methodology of QOL core outcomes measured in BMSC clinical trials. Using descriptive statistics to uncover patterns and counts in the data, the study found that SF36 was the most commonly used instrument; timing/frequency usually was measured at baseline and baseline plus follow-up. Outcomes included disease free survival, disease free intervals, adverse events, quality of life, and psychosocial behavior.

An assessment also was conducted of timing/frequency intervals and methodology of QOL core outcomes measured in cardiovascular stem cell clinical trials and current trials that have not been completed. The most common QOL assessments used in current trials are Rand 36, SF-36, Kansas City Cardiomyopathy, Minnesota Living with Heart Failure, Seattle Angina and EQ-5D.

However, the most common instruments/methodologies implemented were the SF-36, the Minnesota Living with Heart Failure, and EQ-5D. None of the cardiovascular studies BMSC reported QOL at baseline only. The most common follow up was performed post baseline at 6 months or 12 months. The outcomes were consistent depending upon the specific conditions. LVEF changes and decrease in NYHA were most notable outcomes.

A comparison of QOL core outcomes in bone marrow and cardiovascular stem cell clinical trials was measured. BMSC clinical trials outcomes measured disease free survival, disease free interval, adverse events, quality of life, psychosocial behavior, safety, and efficacy, as compared to cardiovascular BMSC outcomes, which focused on LVEF changes and decrease in NYHA classification.

A survey was used to ascertain whether patients were satisfied with the QOL outcomes currently measured in cardiovascular stem cell clinical trials. To investigate, surveys containing six Likert scale questions were sent to patients who had received stem cell treatment and completed a QOL survey. Although the data were limited, they suggested that participants preferred yes/no questions and surveys that required less than 15 minutes to complete. Participants favored email versus web based survey delivery. They responded that the QOL questionnaires administered were easy to understand, not too personal, relevant to their feelings, and specific to their medical conditions. Interestingly, they indicated that a baseline measurement should have been administered.

Interpretation of Findings

Lunde et al. (2005) was the first BMSC clinical trial to include QOL assessment with SF-36; however, they failed to report any QOL results. To further illustrate the problem of not reporting, some researchers captured the QOL data but did not evaluate it and therefore excluded such data from the published results. These findings are useful in that they demonstrate a bias by excluding information vital for determining treatment efficacy in the current literature.

The methodologies used in BMSC cardiovascular trials are country specific. EQ-5D seems to be the preferred methodology choice in European BMSC cardiovascular clinical trials, whereas, the USA uses SF-36, which further illustrates the disparity between countries.

The use of timing/frequency intervals and QOL core outcomes methodology measured in BMSC cardiovascular trials are still in their infancy. In an attempt to have a basis for comparison, the researcher reviewed BMSC clinical trials to identify some type of "gold standard" (Claassen, 2005). For example, as far back as 1990, The National Cancer Institute clinical trial and QOL expert workshop attempted address QOL end-point implementation (Nayfield et al. 1992). Conversely, the study found diverse methodologies, timing/frequency inconsistencies, and outcomes used in the BMSC clinical trials. BMSC clinical trials were consistent when measuring baseline, whereas no cardiac BMSC trials measured baseline. This finding is relevant because it is impossible to determine treatment efficacy without a baseline for comparison. Without QOL assessment, patients cannot give true informed consent, nor can they be fully aware of the full continuum of treatment outcomes. Additionally, QOL assessments augment the clinical decision-making process for the clinician and the patient. Moreover, QOL assessments are the most

44

consistent prognostic factors for post-transplant psychosocial problems.

Research can help develop possible standardization of QOL core outcomes for future cardiovascular stem cell clinical trials. This study is the first of its kind to address this issue. Heart disease is on the rise and new, cost effective QOL measurements must be considered. Furthermore, QOL core outcomes must be taken into account for treatment efficacy. The foundational work of this study supports the need for QOL core outcomes standardization as stem cell clinical trials may produce significant treatment benefits to millions of aging people in a currently overburdened health care system.

Limitations and Strengths of the Study

Study Selection

This study found that QOL outcomes are not routinely included in cardiovascular BMSC trials. Indeed, the very newness of QOL outcomes studies led to a relatively small publications sample. As a result of these factors, the literature review was limited in number of cardiovascular BMSC clinical trials, which made the selection too small for statistical strength.

Patient Survey

The patient survey was administered by email to gain consensus about QOL questionnaires. To minimize bias and peer pressure, other methods such as interview or focus groups were not considered. There were no ethical challenges to address. However, the lack of participant response made the study less statistically powerful. While the study anticipated 15-30 participants for the QOL questionnaire, only ten participants opened the QOL survey, and only four participants completed the entire questionnaire. Some who returned the survey did so without completing all of the questions, leading to missing data. Therefore, the survey sample size and completion rate were inadequate to the study's goals.

Assumptions

One theoretical assumption made was that cancer BMSC clinical trials had a consensus in methodologies, timing/frequency, and outcomes. This foundational base could have been the platform for standardizing QOL outcomes for the cardiovascular BMSC QOL. However, the study discovered that it could not use cancer BMSC as a foundational base because standardized QOL outcomes are needed just as much as cardiovascular BMSC QOL core outcomes.

Lessons Learned

The call for participants was made four times. However, participation was extremely low. In an effort to prevent low participation, the researcher called by telephone and sent emails to over 50 previously treated cardiovascular stem cell patients. Additionally, the researcher used email to contact treating organizations (e.g. Repair Stem Cell, and Regenocell) that have access to hundreds of treated patients, but none responded. In a final attempt to rectify the low response, the researcher contacted the International Cell Medicine Society, a registry that has compiled 750 treated follow up cases; however, they did not have a process that would allow for collecting external data.

Loss of data due to follow up problems and patient noncompliance is a problem as one well-known private stem cell treating company learned after treating several hundred cases. Each patient was administered an SF-36 at baseline on site. At home, each patient received follow up to complete a QOL survey by email at 1, 3, 6 months and 1, 2, 3, 4, and 5 years. The response was very poor and the company assigned qualified personnel to contact each patient more personally. Much time was exhausted contacting each patient for follow up. This experience demonstrated that sending out emails is not enough; it is important to have personal touch to motivate patients to comply with such requests. In retrospect, it would have been interesting to have a consensus from both clinicians and patients. Patient compliance is a problem and in the future one-on-one interview and polling techniques could be useful in order to maximize the population sample.

It is important not to assume that what is perceived is correct. For example, in this study, cancer BMSC was utilized due to its long timeline, thinking that this would be a good foundation for cardiovascular BMSC. However, it proved not to be a good foundation for cardiovascular BMSC. In the future, it is best not to combine such studies as they are not as similar as might be expected.

Furthermore, there may have been more respondents in this study's patient satisfaction survey if participants had not been told that they could stop at any time. Because participants appear to need one-on-one follow up to attain the population sample needed, future studies involving participants should provide that one-on-one experience and/or another incentive to complete the instrument.

CHAPTER 6: RECOMMENDATIONS AND CONCLUSIONS

Recommendations for Further Study

This study revealed the potential for improving BMSC cardiovascular trials in assessment and QOL methodological approaches. Based on the study findings, the inconsistency between multiple QOL rating scales, timing/frequency, and heterogeneity in BMSC clinical trials warrants further evaluation and research.

The COMET Initiative recommendations should be considered as the necessary next step to advance QOL standardization and to establish QOL core outcomes. The Delphi technique could be used to form the consensus for the clinicians, which would reduce bias. From a participant perspective, QOL testing should be initiated prior to treatment for baseline measure, post treatment: 3 months, 6 months, 12 months and 24 months.

Methodologies for cardiovascular BMSC trials should consist of two of three instruments (i.e., SF36 *and* NYHA *or* CCS classification) and a QOL assessment specific to the type of disease (e.g., cardiomyopathy or coronary artery disease). Typically, a heart failure study would use SF-36 and NYHA, while a coronary artery disease study would use SF-36 and CCS for an angina classification. Clinicians may be interested in administering a psychosocial assessment, which could influence QOL results either positively or negatively (Meyers et al. 1994). This type of assessment is valuable if intervention is indicated. QOL importance is evident. If the clinicians do not wish to administer and publish their results, they should consider outsourcing this testing to an independent agency, so that the results can become available.

There also appears to be publication bias in the literature as the majority of the cardiovascular BMSC studies report positive results. Furthermore, some clinical trials capture QOL but do not report results. For example, Roncalli et al. (2010) conducted a QOL assessment but did not have the time to assess and therefore did not publish the data. Even though cardiovascular BMSC consistently use the same QOL methodologies (i.e., SF-36, and/or MLHF), there may be missing data and/or uneven study or reporting of such data as treatment timing, delivery techniques, optimal dosage, and the best cell types. Cardiovascular BMSC trials, for example, do not measure baseline, which means that it cannot be known whether cardiovascular BMSC treatments are effective since there is no baseline measure to compare. In this research, patients expressed that they preferred a baseline measure. Therefore, it is crucial to research and initiate QOL standardization in cardiovascular BMSC clinical trials to set a "gold standard" minimum. This standardization will be vital to physicians and patients in the decision-making process and to give true informed consent.

Conclusion

This study indicates that very few research studies address QOL outcomes for BMSC cardiovascular clinical trials. It demonstrated the need for standardization of core outcomes in cardiovascular BMSC clinical trials. The studies assessed were inconsistent in methodology, timing/frequency, and outcomes. In other words, there is no standardized protocol to evaluate QOL outcomes. Without standards, researchers lack the tools with which to evaluate clinical trials properly and determine treatment efficacy. The disparity and heterogeneity of BMSC cardiovascular clinical trials results in the inability to make evidence-based treatment choices.

Ethically, accountability is jeopardized without QOL standards. Treatments are performed worldwide, and no one knows whether these treatments actually are working. To this end, it is important to utilize programs like the COMET Initiative and to standardize QOL outcomes for cardiovascular stem trials.

1	
	1. I thought the Quality of Life **i. What was the name of the quality of life survey?**

1. I thought the Quality of Life

Too personal
Too complicated
Too time consuming
Too long
Hard to understand

i. What was the name of the quality of life survey?

☐ Short Form 12 (SF-12)
☐ Short Form 36 (SF-36)
☐ Minnesota Heart Scale
☐ Do not know
☐ Other (please specify)

[_____]

2	

3

. I prefer the Quality of Life survey to be administered by

	Strongly disagree	Disagree	Neither	Agree
Telephone	○	○	○	○
Email	○	○	○	○
Office Visit	○	○	○	○
iPad	○	○	○	○
Web-based self-administered	○	○	○	○
Other (please specify)				

[_____]

4

. I think Quality of Life survey should be administered

	Strongly disagree	Disagree	Neither	Agree
Before treatment	○	○	○	○
During treatment	○	○	○	○
1 month after treatment	○	○	○	○
3 months after treatment	○	○	○	○
6 months after treatment	○	○	○	○
1 year after treatment	○	○	○	○
2 years after treatment	○	○	○	○

5

. I think the Quality of Life questions were relevant to

	Strongly disagree	Disagree	Neither	Agree
My condition	○	○	○	○
My feelings	○	○	○	○
What I was experiencing	○	○	○	○
My emotional well-being	○	○	○	○

6

I would prefer to complete a Quality of Life questionnaire provided it took

	Strongly disagree	Disagree	Neither	Agree
10 minutes	○	○	○	○
15 minutes	○	○	○	○
30 minutes	○	○	○	○
60 minutes	○	○	○	○

7

. I prefer this format when answering questionaires

	Strongly disagree	Disagree	Neither	Agree
One answer (Yes/no)	○	○	○	○
Multiple Choice (multiple answers)	○	○	○	○
Essay /Comments	○	○	○	○
Rating Scale (1, 2, 3, 4, 5)	○	○	○	○

8	. Tell us about yourself	
	Gender	
	Highest degree	
	Age	
	City/Town:	
	State:	– select state –
	ZIP:	
	Country:	

Title
Standardization of Quality of Life Core Outcomes in Stem Cell Clinical Trials
Introduction and background
Establishing standardized Quality of Life (QOL) core outcomes in stem cell clinical trials is important to ensure that 1) researchers and clinicians can make informed decisions, and 2) clinical trials are using the same units, and measuring those units in the same way (Clarke, 2007; see also Thornley & Adams, 1998). Standardisation of outcomes is also important because, according to COMET (Core Outcome Measures in Effectiveness Trials), it makes "it easier to compare, contrast and synthesize" clinical trial outcomes, while reducing bias and incongruity (University of Liverpool, 2010). However, before core outcomes in stem cell clinical trials can be established, a necessary first step is to describe and evaluate the QOL core outcomes currently in use.   To date, some research has been conducted in the area of bone marrow stem cell (BMSC) clinical trials, however, a dearth of standardised QOL core outcome measurements in the area of cardiovascular clinical trials remains. Therefore, this study intends to identify QOL core outcomes currently being measured for both BMSC and cardiovascular stem cell clinical trials, more specifically the timing / frequency and methodology of those outcomes being measured. Furthermore, using the COMET initiative as a guide, this study will evaluate the potential for using standardised core outcomes. BMSC and cardiovascular stem cell clinical trial treatment outcomes will be compared and contrasted, in addition to measuring patient satisfaction. The purpose of this study is to evaluate and explore the possibility of standardising QOL core outcomes in cardiovascular stem cell trials by using BMSC as a base framework.
Literature Summary
There are a number of issues related to standardising outcomes, particularly in the field of clinical trial stem cell research. One issue is the timing/frequency intervals in which outcomes are measured. According to Packman, et al. (2010), BMSC QOL outcomes are typically measured pre, during, and post transplant, regardless of the number of months transpiring. In contrast, a cardiovascular stem cell FOCUS study measured QOL outcomes post treatment at 3, 6, and 12-month intervals (Willerson, et al. 2010). Thus, 'time' at which the QOL tool is administered is not taken into account in both frameworks. Furthermore, the Willerson study (2010) lacked a QOL baseline whereas Packman, et al. (2010) had a baseline to compare pre-intervention outcomes, yet secondary endpoints were measured subjectively by using the New York Heart Association (NYHA) and Canadian Cardiovascular Society functional classifications. This is an important point because we do not know if the patient was the same, better, or worse after one year prior to having the

transplant. Due to these variations, non-standardisation of QOL outcomes in regards to timing/frequency intervals and instruments used makes it difficult to analyze whether QOL has improved or declined from study to study. Therefore, it is necessary to understand when and how QOL outcomes are currently being measured in stem cell clinical trials, and what potential standardisations can be proposed.

Additionally, another area of consideration regarding the standardisation of QOL outcomes in stem cell clinical trials pertains to the actual tool or instrument being used for measuring outcomes (Mosher, 2010; Le, et al., 2010; and Slovacek, 2007). Even outside of the field of stem cell research we can see the need for standardisation as evidenced by the Thornlay and Adams' (1998) study of 2000 controlled trials in schizophrenia over a 50 year period, where they found more than 600 different rating scales used, leading to a lack of statistical power. This further illustrates the need for creating a core set of outcomes per disease or condition-specific clinical trials. The current study aims to explore this need.

Research Question (RQ)

What are the quality of life core outcomes currently being measured in stem cell clinical trials?

Aim & objectives

Aim: To describe and evaluate the quality of life core outcomes currently being measured in stem cell clinical trials.

Objectives:

Describe the timing / frequency intervals, and methodology of QOL core outcomes being measured in bone marrow stem cell clinical trials.

Describe the timing / frequency intervals, and methodology of QOL core outcomes being measured in cardiovascular stem cell clinical trials.

Compare and contrast QOL core outcomes measured in both groups (bone marrow and cardiovascular stem cell clinical trials).

Assess patient satisfaction with the QOL outcomes that are currently being measured in cardiovascular stem cell clinical trials.

Explore possible standardisation of QOL core outcomes in cardiovascular stem cell clinical trials.

Methods

Literature Review

This will be a contrastive literature review of QOL outcomes in bone marrow and cardiovascular stem cell clinical trials.

Search Strategy - Inclusion Criteria:

Review stem cell transplant clinical trials that include QOL.

Literature review will focus on studies conducted from 2000-2010. The reason this study will focus on this timeframe is due to the dearth of stem cell research prior to 2005 except for BMSC transplants in cancer patients. An initial search of available citations revealed the following:

Results from Scopus:

bone marrow stem cell transplant =6,680

bone marrow stem cell transplant + quality of life=152

bone marrow stem cell + quality of life= 681

bone marrow stem cell + heart=3,382

bone marrow stem cell + cardiac=1,641

bone marrow stem cell + cardiac+ QOL=27

Results from Clinical Trial.gov,

bone marrow stem cells=1409

bone marrow stem cells + QOL=86

Results from Medline

bone marrow stem cell AND quality of life (Broad search) =194

bone marrow stem cell AND quality of life (Narrow search) =14

bone marrow stem cell AND cardiac AND quality of life=4

Relevant materials search including, but not limited to, libraries catalogues, databases, internet, and bibliographies.

Language restriction: English.

Research terms will include:

Stem cell transplantation AND QOL

Hematopoietic stem cell transplantation AND QOL

Bone marrow stem cell AND QOL

Cardiac, heart and cardiovascular stem cell transplant

Cardiac, heart and cardiovascular stem cell transplant AND QOL

Literature Review Exclusion Criteria:

The exclusion criteria included all works that are unpublished in peer-reviewed journal, i.e. conference papers, master's theses, doctoral dissertations, and unpublished working papers.

QOL Survey

The study will include a Likert scale web-based questionnaire comprised of eight questions designed to assess patient satisfaction with outcomes currently being measured as part of cardiovascular stem cell clinical trials as determined by the literature review.

The anticipated number of participants in this part of the study is 15-30. The samples from the Stem Cell Pioneer board are primarily US-based and located in urban areas. The population group will be diverse. Patients will be recruited voluntarily by two methods:

A recruitment message for study volunteers will be posted to the Stem Cell Pioneers Board. The message will explain that qualified participants (patients previously treated with autologous stem cells) are being sought for a Quality of Life Study investigating how outcomes are measured. Those interested will be asked to contact the student investigator by email. The potential participants will then be screened for eligibility by a brief telephone call.

A random sampling of previously treated patients from a private autologous stem cell company will be drawn from a list, contacted by email, and invited to participate in the study. These participants also must meet the eligibility requirements outlined.

Eligibility requirements include that participants must be 18-75 years of age, post-autologous stem cell treatment patients and were administered QOL questionnaires.

Following the administration of the questionnaire, all data will be coded, verified, and analyzed as percentages. The   will be used for comparing the two groups collected from the Likert scale.

The researcher will seek either written consent agreements or digitally recorded permission statements to protect participants' confidentiality. Both a Research Ethics application form and necessary accompanying documentation will be sent to University of Liverpool. An information sheet and a consent form will be incorporated into the survey so that participants may acknowledge their informed consent.

Research Outcomes

Research outcomes will 1) assess the potential for standardising QOL outcome in cardiovascular stem cell transplant studies 2) consider a model of standardisation for general stem cell treatment outcomes.

Costs

The total cost of this study will be minimal. Costs include telephone calls using the researcher's telephone, the researcher's own time, and the use of a free- or low-cost web-based survey tool like SurveyMonkey or Zoomerang. The greatest cost factor would be the researcher's time spent in analyzing and synthesizing the data.

Timetable

The researcher's goal is to complete all chapters equalling the first thesis draft at least two months before it is due for submission.
MONTH 2: DA/Student agreement 'sign off'
MONTH 3: Submit improved questions to DA
MONTH 4: Submit draft introductory chapter to DA
MONTH 5: Data collection and initial analysis

MONTH 6: Data collection and initial analysis
MONTH 7: Submit draft Methodology and Results chapters to DA by end of month.
MONTH 8: Submit draft discussion chapter to DA
MONTH 9: Final draft to DA for review by end of the month
MONTH 10: Final Dissertation to be submitted

References

Le, R.Q., Bevans, M., Savani, B.N., Mitchell, S.A., Stringaris, K., Koklanaris, E. & Barrett, A.J. (2010) "Favorable Outcomes in Patients Surviving 5 or More Years after Allogeneic Hematopoietic Stem Cell Transplantation for Hematologic Malignancies", *Biology of Blood and Marrow Transplantation,* vol. 16, no. 8, pp. 1162-1170. [Online]. DOI:10.1016/j.bbmt.2010.03.005 (Accessed: 1 October 2010).

Mosher, C.E., DuHamel, K.N., Rini, C., Corner, G., Lam, J. & Redd, W.H. (2010) "Quality of life concerns and depression among hematopoietic stem cell transplant survivors", *Supportive Care in Cancer,* , pp. 1-9. [Online]. Available from: http://www.springerlink.com.ezproxy.liv.ac.uk/content/6588043573n28224/fulltext.pdf (Accessed 1 October 2010).

Packman, S., Weber, J., Wallace and N Bugescu (2010) Bone Marrow Transplantation 45, 1134–1146 [Online],. Available from: http://www.nature.com.ezproxy.liv.ac.uk/bmt/journal/v45/n7/pdf/bmt201074a.pdf (Accessed: 30 September 2010).

Slovacek, L., Slovackova, B., Pavlik, V., and Jebavy, L. (2007) Health-related quality of life in acute myeloid leukaemia and multiple myeloma survivors undergoing autologous progenitor stem cell transplantation: a retrospective analysis, Reports of Practical Oncology & Radiotherapy, Volume 12, Issue 4, July-August 2007, Pages 231-238, [Online] Available from: (http://www.sciencedirect.com/science/article/B9HCH-4YR97GD-6/2/73ddfeb844924e3a873b9b4ecd593950) (Accessed: 1 October 2010) .

Thornley, B., and Adams C. (1998) BMJ. 1998 Oct 31;317(7167):1181-4. [Online]. Available from: http://www.ncbi.nlm.nih.gov/pmc/articles/PMC28699/ (Accessed: 2 October 2010)

UoL (2010) COMET Initiative [Online] Available from: http://www.liv.ac.uk/nwhtmr/research/theme_2/core_outcomes.htm (Accessed: 30 September 2010).

Willerson, J.T. , Perin , E.C., Ellis, S.G., Pepine, C.J., Henry, T.D., Zhao, D.X.M., Lai, D., Penn, M.S., Byrne, B.J., Silva, G., Gee, A., Traverse, J.H., Hatzopoulos, A.K., Forder, J.R., Martin, D., Kroenberg, M., Taylor, D.A., Cogle, C.R., Baraniuk, S., Westbrook, L., Sayre, S.L., Vojuvodic, R.W., Gordon, D.J., Skarlatos, S.I., Moye, L.A. & Simari, R.D. (2010). Intramyocardial injection of autologous bone marrow mononuclear cells for patients with chronic ischemic heart disease and left ventricular dysfunction (First Mononuclear Cells injected in the US [FOCUS]): Rationale and design. *American Heart Journal,* **160**(2), 215-223. [Online]. Available from: http://www.sciencedirect.com/science/article/B6W9H-50PKK8G-5/2/5204f41fa6f0224de75fea9a46eb65b7 (Accessed: 1 October 2010).

REFERENCES

American Heart Association (2011a) *Heart Transplants: Statistics* [Online]. Available from: http://www.americanheart.org/presenter.jhtml?identifier=4588 (Accessed: 9 June 2011).

Andrykowski,M.A., Greiner,C.B., Altmaier,E.M., Burish,T.G., Antin,J.H., Gingrich,R., McGanrgle,C., & Henslee-Downey, P.J. (1995) 'Quality of life following bone marrow transplantation: findings from a multicentre study' *British Journal of Cancer* 71, 1322-1329 [Online]. Available from: http://www.ncbi.nlm.nih.gov/pmc/articles/PMC2033838/pdf/brjcancer00052-0202.pdf (Accessed: 26 February 2011).

Bundkirchen, A. & Schwinger, R.H.G. (2004) 'Epidemiology and economic burden of chronic heart failure', *Eur Heart J Suppl*, 6(suppl D): D57-D60 [Online]. DOI:10.1016/j.ehjsup.2004.05.015 (Accessed: 30 November 2010).

Beeken, R.J., Eiser, C., & Dalley. C. (2010) Health-related quality of life in haematopoietic stem cell transplant survivors: a qualitative study on the role of psychosocial variables and response shifts Qual Life Res [Online]. DOI 10.1007/s11136-010-9737-y (Accessed: 6 December 2010).

BMJ Blogs (2011a) 'Quality' more important than 'quantity' at end of life, [Online/ Blog]. Available from: http://blogs.bmj.com/spcare/2011/03/29/individuals-place-greater-value-on-quality-than-quantity-at-end-of-life/ (Accessed: 7 April 2011).

BMJ Blogs (2010b) Comet Initiative, [Online/ Blog]. Available from: http://blogs.bmj.com/bmj/2010/03/08/the-comet-initiative/ (Accessed: 20 January 2010).

CDC (2010a) *Health related quality of life* [Online]. Available from: http://www.cdc.gov/hrqol/ (Accessed: 9 February 2011).

CDC (2010b) *Heart Disease Facts* [Online]. Available from: http://www.cdc.gov/heartdisease/facts.htm (Accessed: 27 January 2011).

Cella,D.F. (1994) 'Quality of life: Concepts and definition', *Journal of Pain and Symptom Management*, Volume 9, Issue 3, Pages 186-192, [Online]. DOI: 10.1016/0885-3924(94)90129-5 (Accessed: 28 January 2011).

Claassen, J (2005) 'The gold standard: not a golden standard', *BMJ* 330:1121 [Online]. Available from: http://www.bmj.com/content/330/7500/1121.full#cited-by (Accessed: 30 January 2011).

Clarke, M. (2007) 'Standardising outcomes for clinical trials and systematic reviews', Trials 2007, 8:39 [Online]. DOI: 10.1186/1745-6215-8-39. (Accessed: 30 September 2010).

Coyne, K.S., & Allen, J.K. (1998) 'Assessment of functional status in patients with cardiac disease', *Heart & Lung: The Journal of Acute and Critical Care* Vol. 27, Issue 4, Pages 263-273 [Online]. Available from: http://www.sciencedirect.com/science?_ob=MImg&_imagekey=B6WG7-4CNT29H-43-1&_cdi=6815&_user=8554888&_pii=S0147956398900383&_origin=search&_zone=rslt_list_item&_coverDate=08%2F31%2F1998&_sk=999729995&wchp=dGLzVlb-zSkzV&md5=ebbed0cf6c688c8730e2bcd7f4c2fa05&ie=/sdarticle.pdf (Accessed: 27 February 2011).

Creswell, J. (2003). Research design: Qualitative, quantitative, and mixed methods approaches. New York NY: Sage Publications, Inc.

Dalkey, N. (1968) The Delphi Technique: An Experimental Study of Group Opinion [Online]. Available from: http://www.rand.org/content/dam/rand/pubs/research_memoranda/2005/RM5888.pdf (Accessed: 9 June 2011).

Donald, A. (2003) *What is Quality of Life*. [Online]. Available from: http://www.whatisseries.co.uk/whatis/pdfs/What_is_QOL.pdf Available from: (Accessed: 30 November 2010).

European Heart Network (2009) *Annual Reports*, [Online]. Available from: http://www.ehnheart.org/publications/annual-reports.html (Accessed: 25 June 2011).

Fox Chase Cancer Center (2007) *Quality of Life is the Most Important Indicator for Predicting Survival of Patients With Advanced Non-Small Cell Lung Cancer* [Online]. Available from: http://www.fccc.edu/news/2007/Nicolaou-ASTRO-10-30-07.html (Accessed: 2 January 2011).

Heron, M.P., Hoyert, D.L,. Murphy, S.L., Xu, J.Q., Kochanek, K.D., Tejada-Vera, B. (2009) Deaths: Final data for 2006. [Online]. Available from: http://www.cdc.gov/nchs/data/nvsr/nvsr57/nvsr57_14.pdf (Accessed: 27 January 2011).

Hjermstad & Kaasa (1995). "Quality of Life in Adult Cancer Patients Treated with Bone: Marrow Transplantation–a Review of the Literature", *European Journal of Cancer*, Vol. 31A, No. 2, pp. 163-173 [Online]. DOI:10.1016/0959-8049(94)00464-G (Accessed: 27 February 2011).

Hughes, S. (2004) BOOST study published: An "important first" for stem-cell research and the heart [Online]. Available from: http://www.theheart.org/article/148671.do#bib_3 (Accessed: 10 June 2011).

JAMA (2002) 'JAMA Patient Quality of Life', *JAMA* 288(23):3070. [Online]. DOI:10.1001/jama.288.23.3070 (Accessed: 9 February 2011).

King College London (2011), *BRIEFING NOTE Survey of public priorities for end-of-life care across Europe*[Online]. Available from: http://www.kcl.ac.uk/newsevents/publications/SurveyResults.pdf (Accessed: 7 April 2011).

Le, R.Q., Bevans, M., Savani, B.N., Mitchell, S.A., Stringaris, K., Koklanaris, E. and Barrett, A.J. (2010) 'Favorable Outcomes in Patients Surviving 5 or More Years after Allogeneic Hematopoietic Stem Cell Transplantation for Hematologic Malignancies', *Biology of Blood and Marrow Transplantation*, vol. 16, no. 8, pp. 1162-1170. [Online]. DOI:10.1016/j.bbmt.2010.03.005 (Accessed: 1 October 2010).

Lunde, K., Solheim, S., Aakhus, S, Arnesen, H., Abdelnoor, M. & Forfang, K. (2005) 'Autologous stem cell transplantation in acute myocardial infarction: The ASTAMI randomized controlled trial. Intracoronary transplantation of autologous mononuclear bone marrow cells, study design and safety aspects', *Scandinavian Cardiovascular Journal* 39: 150/158 [Online]. DOI: 10.1080/14017430510009131 (Accessed: 9 February 2011).

Martin, D. (2010) *Dr. Georges Mathé, Transplant Pioneer, Dies at 88*, The New York Times, Research, [Online] Available from: http://www.nytimes.com/2010/10/21/health/research/21mathe.html?_r=1 (Accessed: 27 October 2010).

Mathur, A & Martin J.F.(2004)'Stem cells and repair of the heart', *The Lancet*, Volume 364 Issue 9429 Pages 183-192 [Online] DOI: 10.1016/S0140-6736(04)16632-4) (Accessed: 15 June 2011).

Meyers C.A. et al. (1994) 'Evaluation of the neurobehavioral functioning of patients before, during, and after bone marrow transplantation'. *J Clin Oncol* 12: [Online]. Available from: http://jco.ascopubs.org/content/12/4/820.abstract (Accessed: 2 January 2011).

Morrison, M., & Samwick, A. A. (1940) 'Intramedullary (sternal) transfusion of human bone marrow', *J Am Med Assoc.*1940;115:1708–1711 [Online] DOI: 10.1001/jama.1940.02810460040010

MRC (2010) *COMET Initiative* [Online]. Available from: http://www.methodologyhubs.mrc.ac.uk/news__events/comet_initiative.aspx (Accessed: 28 January 2011).

Mosher, C.E., DuHamel, K.N., Rini, C., Corner, G., Lam, J. and Redd, W.H. (2010) 'Quality of life concerns and depression among hematopoietic stem cell transplant survivors', *Supportive

Care in Cancer, , pp. 1-9. [Online]. Available from:
http://www.springerlink.com.ezproxy.liv.ac.uk/content/6588043573n28224/fulltext.pdf
(Accessed 1 October 2010).

Muldoon, M. F., Barger, S. D., Flory, J. D. & Manuck, S. B. (1998) 'What are quality of life
measurements measuring?' *B.M.J.* 316: 542-545 [Online]. Available from:
http://www.bmj.com/content/316/7130/542.abstract#cited-by (Accessed: 5 January 2011).

Murphy, M.K., Black, N.A., Lamping, D.L., McKee, C.M., Sanderson, C.F.B., Askham, J. &
Marteau, T. (1998) 'Consensus development methods, and their use in clinical guideline
development: a review', *Health Technology Assessment* 1998; Vol. 2: No. 3 [Online]. DOI:
10.3310/hta2030 (Accessed: 22 February 2011).

Nayfield, S. G., Ganz, P. A., Moinpour, C. M., Cella, D. F., & Hailey, B. J. (1992) 'Report from a
National Cancer Institute (USA) workshop on quality of life assessment in cancer clinical
trials' *Quality of Life Research* Volume 1, Number 3, 203-210, [Online] DOI:
10.1007/BF00635619 (Accessed: 26 February 2011).

Neuman, W. L. (2003). Social research methods (5th edition.). Upper Saddle River, NJ: Prentice
Hall.

Organ Procurement and Transplant Network (2011) National Data, [Online]. Available from:
http://optn.transplant.hrsa.gov/latestData/step2.asp (Accessed: 9 June 2011).

Osgood, E.E., Riddle, M.C., & Mathews, T.J. (1939) 'Aplastic anemia treated with daily transfusions
and intravenous marrow; case report.' *Am J Med.* 1939;13:357–367. [Online]
DOI:10.1059/0003-4819-13-2-357 (Accessed: 18 February 2011).

Packman, S., Weber, J., Wallace and N Bugescu (2010) 'Psychological effects of hematopoietic SCT
on pediatric patients, siblings and parents: a review',*Bone Marrow Transplantation* 45,
1134–1146 [Online],. Available from:
http://www.nature.com.ezproxy.liv.ac.uk/bmt/journal/v45/n7/pdf/bmt201074a.pdf
(Accessed: 30 September 2010).

Patel, A. N., Geffner, L., Vina, R. F., Saslavsky, J., Urschel, H. C., Jr, Kormos, R., and Benetti, F
(2005)
'Surgical treatment for congestive heart failure with autologous adult stem cell
transplantation: A prospective randomized study', *J Thorac Cardiovasc Surg* 130: 1631-
1638 [Online]. DOI: 10.1016/j.jtcvs.2005.07.056 (Accessed: 9 February 2011).

Perin, E. C., Dohmann, H.F.R., Borojevic, R., Silva, S. A., Sousa, A.L.S., Mesquita, C. T., Rossi,
M.I.D.. Carvalho, A.C., Dutra, H.S., Dohmann, H.J.F., Silva, G. V., Belém, L., Vivacqua,
R.,. Rangel, F.O.D., Esporcatte, R.,. Geng, Y.J., Vaughn, W.K., Assad, J.A.R., Mesquita,
E.T. & Willerson, J. T. (2003a) 'Transendocardial, Autologous Bone Marrow Cell

Transplantation for Severe, Chronic Ischemic Heart Failure',
Circulation 107: 2294-2302; [Online]. DOI:10.1161/01.CIR.0000070596.30552.8B
(Accessed: 10 February 2011).

Perin,E.C.,Silva,G.V.,Henry,T.D.,Cabreira-Hansen,M.G.,Moore,W.H., Coulter,S.A.,
Herlihy,J.P.,Fernandes,M.R., Cheong,B.YC., Flamm, S.D., Traverse,J.H., Zheng,Y.,
Smith,D., Shaw,S., Westbrook,L.,Olson,R.,Patel,D., Gahremanpour,A.,
Canales,J.,Vaughn,W.K., Willerson, J.T. (2011b) 'A randomized study of transendocardial
injection of autologous bone marrow mononuclear cells and cell function analysis in
ischemic heart failure (FOCUS-HF),'*American Heart Journal*, Volume 161, Issue 6, June
2011, Pages 1078-1087.e3, ISSN 0002-8703, [Online]. DOI: 10.1016/j.ahj.2011.01.028.
(Accessed: 12 June 2011).

PROMIS (2011) *Access to the generic instruments*, [Online]. Available from:
http://proqolid.org/proqolid/search___1/generic (Accessed:10 January 2011).

Ring, L., Hofer, S., Heuston, F., Harris,D., & O'Boyle, C. (2005) *Response shift masks the treatment
impact on patient reported outcomes (PROs): the example of individual* [Online]. Available
from: http://www.hqlo.com/content/pdf/1477-7525-3-55.pdf (Accessed:10 January 2011).

Roncalli, J., Mouquet, F., Piot, C., Trochu, J.N., Corvoisier, P.L., Neuder, Y., Tourneau, T.L.,
Agostini, D., Gaxotte, V., Sportouch, C., Galinier, M., Crochet, D., Teiger, E., Richard,
M.J., Polge, A.S., Beregi, J.P., Manrique, A., Carrie, D., Susen, S., Klein, B., Parini, A.,
Lamirault, G., Croisille, P., Rouard, H., Bourin, P., Nguyen, J.M., Delasalle, B., Vanzetto,
G., Van Belle, E., & Lemarchand, P. (2010). 'Intracoronary autologous mononucleated
bone marrow cell infusion for acute myocardial infarction: results of the randomized
multicenter BONAMI trial' *Eur Heart J*, ehq455 [Online]. DOI:10.1093/eurheartj/ehq455
(Accessed: 9 February 2011).

Schipper, H. (1983) 'Why Measure Quality of Life', *CAN MED ASSOC J*, vol. 128 no.2, [Online].
Available from:
http://www.ncbi.nlm.nih.gov/pmc/articles/PMC1875788/pdf/canmedaj01393-0062.pdf
(Accessed: 15 November 2010).

Schächinger, V., Erbs, S., Elsässer, A., Haberbosch, W., Hambrecht, R., Hölschermann, H., Yu, J.,
Corti, R., Mathey, D.G., Hamm, C.W., Süselbeck, T., Assmus, B., Tonn, T., Dimmeler, S.,
& Zeiher, A. M. (2006) 'Intracoronary Bone Marrow–Derived Progenitor Cells in Acute
Myocardial Infarction', *New England Journal of Medicine*, 355:1210-1221 [Online] DOI:
10.1056/NEJMoa060186 (Accessed: 14 February 2011).

Silva,G.V., Perin, E.C., Dohmann, H.F., Borojevic, R., Silva, S.A., Sousa, A.L., Assad, J.A.,
Vaughn, W.K., Mesquita, C.T., Belém, L., Carvalho, A.C., Dohmann, H.J., Barroso do
Amaral, E., Coutinho,J., Branco, R., Oliveira, E., & Willerson, J.T. (2004) 'Catheter-based
transendocardial delivery of autologous bone-marrow-derived mononuclear cells in
patients listed for heart transplantation' *Tex Heart Inst J* 31(3):214–9. [Online]. Available

from: http://www.ncbi.nlm.nih.gov/pmc/articles/PMC521759/ (Accessed: 7 February 2011).

Sinha, I.P., Smyth,R.L., & Williamson, P.R. (2011) 'Using the Delphi Technique to Determine Which Outcomes to Measure in Clinical Trials: Recommendations for the Future Based on a Systematic Review of Existing Studies', *PLoS Med* 8(1): e1000393. [Online] DOI:10.1371/journal.pmed.1000393 (Accessed: 21 February 2011).

Slovacek, L., Slovackova, B., Pavlik, V., and Jebavy, L. (2007) 'Health-related quality of life in acute myeloid leukaemia and multiple myeloma survivors undergoing autologous progenitor stem cell transplantation: a retrospective analysis', *Reports of Practical Oncology & Radiotherapy*, Volume 12, Issue 4, July-August 2007, Pages 231-238, [Online] Available from: (http://www.sciencedirect.com/science/article/B9HCH-4YR97GD-6/2/73ddfeb844924e3a873b9b4ecd593950) (Accessed: 1 October 2010) .

Strauer, B.E., Brehm, M., Zeus, T., Köstering, M., Hernandez, A., Sorg, R. V., Kögler, G. & Wernet, P. (2002)
'Repair of Infarcted Myocardium by Autologous Intracoronary Mononuclear Bone Marrow Cell Transplantation in Humans', *Circulation* 106: 1913 - 1918. [Online]. Available from: http://circ.ahajournals.org/cgi/reprint/106/15/1913 (Accessed: 14 February 2011).

Testa, M.A., & Simonson, D. C, (1996) 'Assessment of Quality-of-Life Outcomes' *N Engl J Med* 334:835-840 [Online]. Available from: http://www.nejm.org/doi/pdf/10.1056/NEJM199603283341306 (Accessed: 15 December 2010).

Thomas, D.E., (1990) *Bone Marrow Transplantation-Past, Present and Future*, Nobel Lecture, [Online]. Available from: http://nobelprize.org/nobel_prizes/medicine/laureates/1990/thomas-lecture.pdf (Accessed: 18 February 2011).

Thornley, B., and Adams C. (1998) BMJ. 1998 Oct 31;317(7167):1181-4. [Online]. Available from: http://www.ncbi.nlm.nih.gov/pmc/articles/PMC28699/ (Accessed: 2 October 2010).

United Network for Organ Sharing (2011) Transplant Trends, [Online]. Available from: http://www.unos.org/index.php (Accessed: 9 June 2011).

University of Liverpool (2010) *COMET Initiative* [Online]. Available from: http://www.liv.ac.uk/nwhtmr/research/theme_2/core_outcomes.htm (Accessed: 20 January 2010).

University of Minnesota (2010) *Minnesota Living With Heart Failure Questionnaire* [Online]. Available from: http://www.license.umn.edu/Products/Minnesota-Living-With-Heart-Failure-Questionnaire__Z94019.aspx (Accessed: 30 January 2011).

Wei H M, Wong P, Hsu L F, Shim W (2009) 'Human bone marrow-derived adult stem cells for post-myocardial infarction cardiac repair: current status and future directions', *Singapore Med J Review* 50(10) : 935 [Online]. Available from: http://smj.sma.org.sg/5010/5010ra1.pdf (Accessed: 8 February 2011).

WHO (1948a) *Preamble to the Constitution of the World Health Organization,* as adopted by the International Health Conference, New York, USA [Online]. Available from:http://whqlibdoc.who.int/hist/official_records/constitution.pdf (Accessed: 15 December 2010).

WHO (1997b) *Measuring Quality of Life* [Online]. Available from: http://www.who.int/mental_health/media/68.pdf (Accessed: 9 February 2011).

Willerson, J.T. , Perin , E.C., Ellis, S.G., Pepine, C.J., Henry, T.D., Zhao, D.X.M., Lai, D., Penn, M.S., Byrne, B.J., Silva, G., Gee, A., Traverse, J.H., Hatzopoulos, A.K., Forder, J.R., Martin, D., Kroenberg, M., Taylor, D.A., Cogle, C.R., Baraniuk, S., Westbrook, L., Sayre, S.L., Vojuvodic, R.W., Gordon, D.J., Skarlatos, S.I., Moye, L.A. and Simari, R.D. (2010) 'Intramyocardial injection of autologous bone marrow mononuclear cells for patients with chronic ischemic heart disease and left ventricular dysfunction (First Mononuclear Cells injected in the US [FOCUS]): Rationale and design', *American Heart Journal,* 160(2), 215-223. [Online]. Available from: http://www.sciencedirect.com/science/article/B6W9H-50PKK8G-5/2/5204f41fa6f0224de75fea9a46eb65b7 (Accessed: 1 October 2010).

Wulff. H. (1999) 'The two cultures of medicine: objective facts versus subjectivity and values', *J R Soc Med* 1999;92: 549-52 [Online]. Available from: http://www.ncbi.nlm.nih.gov/pmc/articles/PMC1297426/pdf/jrsocmed00003-0007.pdf (Accessed: 15 November 2010).

Wollert,K.C., Meyer,G.P., Lotz,J., Lichtenberg,S.R., Lippolt,P., Breidenbach,C., Fichtner,S., Korte, T., Hornig,B., Messinger,D., Arseniev,L., Hertenstein,B., Ganser,A., & Drexler,H. (2004) 'Intracoronary autologous bone-marrow cell transfer after myocardial infarction: the BOOST randomised controlled clinical trial', *The Lancet,*Volume 364 Issue 9429 Pages 141-148[Online].DOI: 10.1016/S0140-6736(04)16626-9)(Accessed: 10 February 2011).

Wulff, H. (1999) 'The two cultures of medicine: objective facts versus subjectivity and values', *Journal of Royal Society of Medicine,* Volume 92 [Online]. Available from: http://www.ncbi.nlm.nih.gov/pmc/articles/PMC1297426/pdf/jrsocmed00003-0007.pdf (Accessed: 15 November 2010).

Yousef, M., Schannwell, C.M., Köstering,M., Zeus, T., Brehm, M & Strauer, B.E. (2009) 'The BALANCE Study: Clinical Benefit and Long-Term Outcome After Intracoronary Autologous Bone Marrow Cell Transplantation in Patients with Acute Myocardial Infarction', *J Am Coll Cardiol* 53;2262-2269 [Online]. DOI: 10.1016/j.jacc.2009.02.051 (Accessed: 11 February 2011).

BIBLIOGRAPHY

Alduaij, W. & Illidge, T.M. (2009). Radioimmunotherapy: Strategies for the future in indolent and aggressive lymphoma. *Current oncology reports, 11*(5), 363-370.

Anderlini, P. & Champlin, R. (2002). Use of filgrastim for stem cell mobilisation and transplantation in high-dose cancer chemotherapy. *Drugs, 62*(SUPPL. 1), 79-88.

Anderson, F.S., Kunin-Batson, A.S., Perkins, J.L. &Baker, K.S.(2008). White versus gray matter function as seen on neuropsychological testing following bone marrow transplant for acute leukemia in childhood. *Neuropsychiatric Disease and Treatment, 4* (1 B), 283-288.

Anderson, K.C., Alsina, M., Bensinger, W., Biermann, J.S., Chanan-Khan, A., Cohen, A.D., Devine, S., Djulbegovic, B., Gasparetto, C., Huff, C.A., Jagasia, M., Medeiros, B.C., Meredith, R., Raje, N., Schriber, J., Singhal, S., Somlo, G., Stockerl-Goldstein, K., Tricot, G., Vose, J.M., Weber, D., Yahalom, J. & Yunus, F. (2009). Multiple myeloma. *JNCCN Journal of the National Comprehensive Cancer Network, 7* (9), 908-942.

Andrykowski, M.A., Bishop, M.M., Hahn, E.A., Cella, D.F., Beaumont, J.L., Brady, M.J., Horowitz, M.M., Sobocinski, K.A., Rizzo, J.D. & Wingard, J.R. (2005). Long-term health-related quality of life, growth, and spiritual well-being after hematopoietic stem-cell transplantation. *Journal of Clinical Oncology, 23* (3), 599-608.

Aurora, V. & Winter, J.N. (2006). Current controversies in follicular lymphoma. *Blood reviews, 20* (4), 179-200.

Aversa, F., Terenzi, A., Felicini, R., Tabilio, A., Falzetti, F., Carotti, A., Falcinelli, F., Sodani, P., Amici, A., Zucchetti, P., Mazzarino, I. & Martelli, M.F. (1998). Mismatched T cell-depleted hematopoietic stem cell transplantation for children with high-risk acute leukemia. *Bone Marrow Transplantation, 22* (Suppl 5), S29-32.

Aversa, F., Terenzi, A., Felicini, R., Tabilio, A., Falzetti, F., Carotti, A., Falcinelli, F., Sodani, P., Amici, A., Zucchetti, P., Mazzarino, I. & Martelli, M.F. (1997). Mismatched T cell-depleted hematopoietic stem cell transplantation for children with high-risk acute leukemia. *Bone Marrow Transplantation, 21*(SUPPL. 5), S29-S32.

Bacigalupo, A., Lamparelli, T., Gualandi, F., Bregante, S., Raiola, A.M., Di Grazia, C., Dominietto, A., Bruno, B., Galbusera, V., Frassoni, F., Podesta, M., Tedone, E., Occhini, D. & Van Lint, M.T. (2002). Prophylactic antithymocyte globulin reduces the risk of chronic graft-versus-host disease in alternative-donor bone marrow transplants. *Biology of Blood and Marrow Transplantation, 8* (12), 656-661.

Baker, K.S., Bresters, D. & Sande, J.E. (2010). The burden of cure: Long-term side effects following Hematopoietic Stem Cell Transplantation (HSCT) in children. *Pediatric clinics of North America, 57*(1), 323-342.

Ballestrero, A., Cirmena, G., Dominietto, A., Garuti, A., Rocco, I., Cea, M., Moran, E., Nencioni, A., Miglino, M., Raiola, A.M., Bacigalupo, A. & Patrone, F. (2010). Peripheral blood vs. bone marrow for molecular monitoring of BCR-ABL1 levels in chronic myelogenous leukemia, a retrospective analysis in allogeneic bone marrow recipients. *International Journal of Laboratory Hematology, 32* (4), 387-391.

Beitinjaneh, A., Burns, L.J. & Majhail, N.S. 2010. Solid organ transplantation in survivors of hematopoietic cell transplantation: A single institution case series and literature review. *Clinical transplantation, 24* (4), E94-E102.

Bellm, L.A., Epstein, J.B., Rose-Ped, A., Martin, P. & Fuchs, H.J. (2000). Patient reports of complications of bone marrow transplantation. *Supportive Care in Cancer, 8* (1), 33-39.

Berger, J.A. (2001). Living The Discipline on a stem cell transplant unit: spiritual care outcomes among bone marrow transplant survivors. *Journal of Health Care Chaplaincy, 11* (1), 83-93.

Bernstein, S.H., Nademanee, A.P., Vose, J.M., Tricot, G., Fay, J.W., Negrin, R.S., Dipersio, J., Rondon, G., Champlin, R., Barnett, M.J., Cornetta, K., Herzig, G.P., Vaughan, W., Geils Jr., G., Keating, A., Messner, H., Wolff, S.N., Miller, K.B., Linker, C., Cairo, M., Hellmann, S., Ashby, M., Stryker, S. & Nash, R.A. (1998). A multicenter study of platelet recovery and utilization in patients after myeloablative therapy and hematopoietic stem cell transplantation. *Blood, 91* (9), 3509-3517.

Bhatia, S., Robison, L.L., Francisco, L., Carter, A., Liu, Y., Grant, M., Baker, K.S., Fung, H., Gurney, J.G., Mcglave, P.B., Nademanee, A., Ramsay, N.K.C., Stein, A., Weisdorf, D.J. & Forman, S.J. (2005). Late mortality in survivors of autologous hematopoietic-cell transplantation: Report from the bone marrow transplant survivor study. *Blood, 105* (11), 4215-4222.

Björkstrand, B. & Gahrton, G. (2007). High-dose treatment with autologous stem cell transplantation in multiple myeloma: Past, present, and future. *Seminars in hematology, 44* (4), 227-233.

Brunet, S., De Soria, V.G.G., Sanz, G., Canales, M., Moraleda, J.M., Caballero, D., Ruiz, D., Bargay, J., Parody, R., De La Serna, J., Cabrera, R., Albo, C., Solano, C., Torres, J.P., Lopez, J., Richard, C., Rodriguez, C.S., Alegre, A., De La Rubia, J., Hernandez-Navarro, F., Vallejo, C., Sierra, J., Sanz, M.A., Ranada, M.F., Torres, A.P. & Tomas, J.F. (2001). Allogeneic bone marrow stem cell transplantation (allo-BMT) vs peripheral blood (allo-PBT) in chronic myeloid leukemia (CML): The Spanish experience. *Blood, 98* (11 PART I), 409a-410a.

Bunjes, D. (2001). The current status of T-cell depleted allogeneic stem-cell transplant in adult patients with AML. *Cytotherapy, 3* (3), 175-188.

Bush, N.E., Donaldson, G.W., Haberman, M.H., Dacanay, R. & Sullivan, K.M. (2000). Conditional and unconditional estimation of multidimensional quality of life after hematopoietic stem cell transplantation: A longitudinal follow-up of 415 patients. *Biology of Blood and Marrow Transplantation, 6* (5 A), 576-591.

Byar, K.L., Eilers, J.E. & Nuss, S.L. (2005). Quality of life 5 or more years post-autologous hematopoietic stem cell transplant. *Cancer Nursing, 28* (2), 148-157.

Carlson, L.E. & Macrae, J.H. (2002). Quality of life issues following autologous bone marrow transplantation. *Expert Review of Pharmacoeconomics and Outcomes Research, 2* (2), 129-146.

Carter, J., Raviv, L., Applegarth, L., Ford, J.S., Josephs, L., Grill, E., Sklar, C., Sonoda, Y., Baser, R.E. & Barakat, R.R. (2010). A cross-sectional study of the psychosexual impact of cancer-related infertility in women: third-party reproductive assistance. *Journal of Cancer Survivorship*, 1-11.

Cazzola, M., Anderson, J.E., Ganser, A. & HellströM-Lindberg, E. (1998). A patient-oriented approach to treatment of myelodysplastic syndromes. *Haematologica, 83* (10), 910-935.

Chang, G., Orav, E.J., Tong, M., & Antin, J.H. (2004). Predictors of 1-year survival assessed at the time of bone marrow transplantation. *Psychosomatics, 45* (5), 378-385.

Chatterjee, R., Kottaridis, P.D., Mcgarrigle, H.H. & Linch, D.C. (2002). Management of erectile dysfunction by combination therapy with testosterone and sildenafil in recipients of high-dose therapy for haematological malignancies. *Bone Marrow Transplantation, 29* (7), 607-610.

Chaudhary, P. & Shah, C. (2010). Update on MDS therapy: From famine to feast. *Cardiovascular and Hematological Agents in Medicinal Chemistry, 8* (4), 187-198.

Chen, N., Kao, R.-. & Lin, C.-. (1999). Umbilical cord blood transplantation and cord blood banking. *Tzu Chi Medical Journal, 11* (4), 301-309.

Clarke, S., Eiser, C. & Skinner, R. (2008). Health-related quality of life in survivors of BMT for paediatric malignancy: A systematic review of the literature. *Bone Marrow Transplantation, 42* (2), 73-82.

Colón-Otero, G. (1999). A critical review of new treatments for the myelodysplastic syndromes. *Cancer Research Therapy and Control, 9* (3-4), 281-288.

Cowan, M.J. (1991). Bone marrow transplantation for the treatment of genetic diseases. *Clinical Biochemistry, 24* (4), 375-381.

Crilley, P. & Goldstein, L.J. (1995). Peripheral blood stem cell transplant in breast cancer. *Seminars in Oncology, 22* (3), 238-249.

Da Fonseca, M.A. (1999). Management of mucositis in bone marrow transplant patients. *Journal of Dental Hygiene: JDH / American Dental Hygienists' Association, 73* (1), 17-21.

Damaj, G., Braud, A. & Hermine, O. (2003). Anemia and chemotherapy for hematological malignancies. *Bulletin du Cancer, 90* (4 SPEC. ISS.), S144-S151.

Davies, S.M., Wagner, J.E., Weisdorf, D.J., Shu, X., Blazar, B.R., Enright, H., Mcglave, P.B. & Ramsay, N.K.C. (1996). Unrelated donor bone marrow transplantation for hematological malignancies-current status. *Leukemia and Lymphoma, 23* (3-4), 221-226.

De La Morena, M.T. & Gatti, R.A. (2010). A history of bone marrow transplantation. *Immunology and Allergy Clinics of North America, 30* (1), 1-15.

Di Cocco, P., Bonanni, L., D'angelo, M., Clemente, K., Greco, S., Rizza, V., Mazzotta, C., Scelzo, C., Famulari, A., Pisani, F. & Orlando, G. (2009). Clinical Operational Tolerance After Solid Organ Transplantation. *Transplantation Proceedings, 41* (4), 1278-1282.

Dos Santos, R.R., Soares, M.B.P., & De Carvalho, A.C.C. (2004). Bone marrow cells transplant in the treatment of chronic chagasic cardiomyopathy. *Revista da Sociedade Brasileira de Medicina Tropical, 37* (6), 490-495.

Drachman, D.B., Jones, R.J., & Brodsky, R.A. (2003). Treatment of refractory myasthenia: "Rebooting" with high-dose cyclophosphamide. *Annals of Neurology, 53* (1), 29-34.

Dreyer, Z.E. (2009). Follow-up into adulthood is critically important for survivors of pediatric transplant. *Bone Marrow Transplantation, 43* (6), 433.

Eden, O.B., Birch, J., Bruce, J., Campbell, R.H.A., Gattamaneni, H.R.G., Jenney, M.E.M., Jones, E., Kelsey, A., Lashford, L.S., Stevens, R.F. & Will, A. (1997). Pediatric oncology and hematology in Manchester, England. *Pediatric Hematology and Oncology, 14* (3), 191-197.

Engelhardt, M., Kleber, M., Udi, J., Wsch, R., Spencer, A., Patriarca, F., Knop, S., Bruno, B., Gramatzki, M., Morabito, F., Kropff, M., Neri, A., Sezer, O., Hajek, R., Bunjes, D., Boccadoro, M., Straka, C., Cavo, M., Polliack, A., Einsele, H., & Palumbo, A. (2010). Consensus statement from European experts on the diagnosis, management, and treatment of multiple myeloma: From standard therapy to novel approaches. *Leukemia and Lymphoma, 51* (8), 1424-1443.

Faraci, M., Morreale, G., Boeri, E., Lanino, E., Dallorso, S., Dini, G., Scuderi, F., Cohen, A. & Cappelli, B. (2008). Unrelated HSCT in an adolescent affected by congenital erythropoietic porphyria. *Pediatric Transplantation, 12* (1), 117-120.

Farquhar, C., Basser, R., Marjoribanks, J. & Lethaby, A. (2003). High dose chemotherapy and autologous bone marrow or stem cell transplantation versus conventional chemotherapy for women with early poor prognosis breast cancer. *Cochrane Database of Systematic Reviews, 1.*

Feichtl, R.E., Rosenfeld, B., Tallamy, B., Cairo, M.S. & Sands, S.A. (2010). Concordance of quality of life assessments following pediatric hematopoietic stem cell transplantation. *Psycho-oncology, 19* (7), 710-717.

Felder-Puig, R., Di Gallo, A., Waldenmair, M., Norden, P., Winter, A., Gadner, H., & Topf, R. (2006). Health-related quality of life of pediatric patients receiving allogeneic stem cell or bone marrow transplantation: Results of a longitudinal, multi-center study. *Bone Marrow Transplantation, 38* (2), 119-126.

Ferry, C. & Socié, G. (2003). Bone marrow transplantation for leukemia: Long term outcome. *Bulletin du Cancer, 90* (7), 601-606.

Filipovich, A.H. (1996). Stem cell transplantation from unrelated donors for correction of primary immunodeficiencies. Immunology and Allergy Clinics of North America, 16(2), 377-392.

Filipovich, A.H., Fasth, A., Portal, F., Landais, P., Pelz, C., Murphy, S., Sobocinski, K., Horowitz, M., King, R., Hegland, J., Kollman, C., & Ireland, M. (1999). Correction of primary immunodeficiencies with bone marrow transplantation from unrelated donors. *Cancer Research Therapy and Control, 9* (1-2), 67-71.

Finiewicz, K.J. & Larson, R.A. (1999). Dose-intensive therapy for adult acute lymphoblastic leukemia. *Seminars in Oncology, 26* (1), 6-20.

Foelber, R. (1998). Autologous stem cell transplant plus interleukin-2 for breast cancer: review and nursing management. *Oncology Nursing Forum, 25* (3), 563-568.

Frame, D. (2007). New strategies in controlling drug resistance. *Journal of Managed Care Pharmacy, 13* (8 SUPPL. A), S13-S17.

Fraser, C.J., Bhatia, S., Ness, K., Carter, A., Francisco, L., Arora, M., Parker, P., Forman, S., Weisdorf, D., Gurney, J.G. & Baker, K.S. (2006). Impact of chronic graft-versus-host disease on the health status of hematopoietic cell transplantation survivors: A report from the Bone Marrow Transplant Survivor Study. *Blood, 108* (8), 2867-2873.

Gajewski, J.L., Foote, M., Tietjen, J., Melson, B., Simmons, A., & Champlin, R.E. (2004). Blood and marrow transplantation compensation: Perspective in payer and provider relations. *Biology of Blood and Marrow Transplantation, 10* (7), 427-432.

Gallardo, D., De La Cámara, R., Nieto, J.B., Espigado, I., Iriondo, A., Jiménez-Velasco, A., Vallejo, C., Martín, C., Caballero, D., Brunet, S., Serrano, D., Solano, C., Ribera, J.M., De La Rubia, J. & Carreras, E. (2009). Is mobilized peripheral blood comparable with bone marrow as a source of hematopoietic stem cells for allogeneic transplantation from HLA-identical sibling donors? A case-control study. *Haematologica, 94* (9), 1282-1288.

Gennery, A.R., Dickinson, A.M., Brigham, K., Barge, D., Spickett, G.P., Curtis, A., Spencer, V., Jackson, A., Cavanagh, G., Carter, V., Palmer, P., Flood, T.J., Cant, A.J. & Abinun, M. (2001). CAMPATH-1M T-cell depleted BMT for SCID: Long-term follow-up of 19 children treated 1987-98 in a single center. *Cytotherapy, 3* (3), 221-232.

Gilbert, C.J. (1996). Peripheral blood progenitor cell transplantation for breast cancer: Pharmacoeconomic considerations. *Pharmacotherapy, 16* (3 II), 101S-108S.

Graubner, U.B., Liese, J., & Belohradsky, B.H. (2001). Vaccination. *Klinische Pädiatrie, 213* (SUPPL. 1), A77-A83.

Hacker, E.D. (2003). Quantitative measurement of quality of life in adult patients undergoing bone marrow transplant or peripheral blood stem cell transplant: a decade in review. *Oncology Nursing Forum, 30* (4), 613-629.

Hale, G., Cobbold, S., Novitzky, N., Bunjes, D., Willemze, R., Prentice, H.G., Milligan, D., Mackinnon, S., & Waldmann, H. (2001). CAMPATH-1 antibodies in stem-cell transplantation. *Cytotherapy, 3* (3), 145-164.

Hale, G.A. & Waldmann, H. (1994). Control of graft-versus-host disease and graft rejection by T cell depletion of donor and recipient with Campath-1 antibodies. Results of matched sibling transplants for malignant diseases. *Bone Marrow Transplantation, 13* (5), 597-611.

Hale, G.A. & Phillips, G.L. (2000). Allogeneic stem cell transplantation for the non-Hodgkin's lymphomas and Hodgkin's disease. *Cancer Treatment Reviews, 26* (6), 411-427.

Hann, D.M., Garovoy, N., Finkelstein, B., Jacobsen, P.B., Azzarello, L.M., & Fields, K.K. (1999). Fatigue and quality of life in breast cancer patients undergoing autologous stem cell transplantation: A longitudinal comparative study. *Journal of Pain and Symptom Management, 17* (5), 311-319.

Henry, D. (1997). Haematological toxicities associated with dose-intensive chemotherapy, the role for and use of recombinant growth factors. *Annals of Oncology, 8* (SUPPL. 3), S7-S10.

Ho, P.J., Gibson, J. & Joshua, D.E. (2004). Treatment of multiple myeloma: Current management and new approaches. *American Journal of Cancer, 3* (1), 47-66.

Holler, E. (2007). Risk assessment in haematopoietic stem cell transplantation: GvHD prevention and treatment. *Best Practice and Research: Clinical Haematology, 20* (2), 281-294.

Horwitz, M.E& Sullivan, K.M. (2006). Chronic Graft-Versus-Host Disease. Blood Reviews, 20(1), 15-27.

Howard, D.H., Meltzer, D., Kollman, C., Maiers, M., Logan, B., Gragert, L., Setterholm, M., & Horowitz, M.M. (2008). Use of cost-effectiveness analysis to determine inventory size for a national cord blood bank. *Medical Decision Making, 28 (*2), 243-253.

Hui, C.H., Bardy, P., Hughes, T., Horvath, N., & To, L.B. (2001). Successful salvage of RAEB/AML relapsing early post allograft with FLAG-Ida conditioned mini-allograft: A report of two cases. *Clinical and Laboratory Haematology, 23* (2), 135-138.

Imataki, O., Nakajima, K., Inoue, N., Tamai, Y. & Kawakami, K. (2010). Evaluation of QOL for stem cell transplantation recipients by SF-36 and FACT-BMT: preliminary results of FACT-BMT for Japanese patients. Gan to kagaku ryoho. *Cancer & Chemotherapy, 37* (5), 847-851.

Intragumtornchai, T., Jootar, S., Unganon, A., Swasdikul, D. & Udomprasertgul, V. (1999). Quality of life in Thai patients after bone marrow and peripheral blood stem cell transplantation: A comparison study with patients treated with conventional chemotherapy. *International Journal of Hematology, 70* (3), 181-189.

Kai, S. & Hara, H. (2003). Allogeneic hematopoietic stem cell transplantation. *Therapeutic Apheresis, 7* (3), 285-291.

Kato, S., 2007. Hematopoietic cell transplantation in X-linked adrenoleukodystrophy. *Brain and Nerve, 59* (4), 339-346.

Katzel, J.A., Hari, P., & Vesole, D.H. (2007). Multiple myeloma: Charging toward a bright future. *CA Cancer Journal for Clinicians, 57* (5), 301-318.

Keating, A. (2007). Prospective clinical trials in BMT come of age in the US: The blood and marrow transplant clinical trials network. *Biology of Blood and Marrow Transplantation, 13* (3), 255-256.

Kennedy, G.A., Morton, J., Western, R., Butler, J., Daly, J., & Durrant, S. (2003). Impact of stem cell donation modality on normal donor quality of life: A prospective randomized study. *Bone marrow transplantation, 31* (11), 1033-1035.

Kikuta, A., Ito, M., Mochizuki, K., Akaihata, M., Nemoto, K., Sano, H., & Ohto, H. (2006). Nonmyeloablative stem cell transplantation for nonmalignant diseases in children with severe organ dysfunction. *Bone marrow transplantation, 38* (10), 665-669.

Kim, H.J., Min, W., Cho, B., Eom, K., Kim, S., Kim, Y., Lee, S., Min, C., Cho, S., Lee, J., & Kim, C.-. (2009). Overcoming various comorbidities by G-CSF-primed unmanipulated BM SCT in adult patients with AML. *Bone Marrow Transplantation, 44* (6), 345-351.

Knight, C., Hind, D., Brewer, N. & Abbott, V. (2004). Rituximab (MabThera®) for aggressive non-Hodgkin's lymphoma: Systematic review and economic evaluation. *Health Technology Assessment, 8* (37), iii-48.

Krasuska, M.E., Dmoszyńska, A., Daniluk, J., & Stanisławek, A. (2002). Information needs of the patients undergoing bone marrow transplantation. *Annales Universitatis Mariae Curie-Sklodowska. Sectio D: Medicina, 57* (2), 178-185.

Krasuska, M.E. & Stanisławek, A. (2003). Communication with patients and their families, who undergo bone marrow transplantation. *Annales Universitatis Mariae Curie-Sklodowska.Sectio D: Medicina, 58* (2), 168-173.

Krivit, W. (2002). Stem cell bone marrow transplantation in patients with metabolic storage diseases. *Advances in Pediatrics, 49*, 359-378.

Kumar, L., Verma, R., & Radhakrishnan, V.R. (2010). Recent advances in the management of multiple myeloma. *National Medical Journal of India, 23* (4), 210-218.

Langer, T., Beck, J., Gravou-Apostulatou, C., Lang, P., Handgretinger, R., & Greil, J. (2003). Successful treatment of primary refractory acute myeloid leukemia with megadose stem cell transplantation, bone marrow boost and reduced intensity conditioning avoiding chronic graft vs. host disease and severe late toxicity. *Pediatric Transplantation, 7* (6), 494-496.

Le, R.Q., Bevans, M., Savani, B.N., Mitchell, S.A., Stringaris, K., Koklanaris, E., & Barrett, A.J. (2010). Favorable outcomes in patients surviving 5 or more years after allogeneic hematopoietic stem cell transplantation for hematologic malignancies. Biology *of Blood and Marrow Transplantation, 16* (8), 1162-1170.

Lee, S.J. (2000). Chronic myelogenous leukaemia. *British Journal of Haematology, 111* (4), 993-1009.

Lee, S.J., Cook, E.F., Soiffer, R. & Antin, J.H. (2002). Development and validation of a scale to measure symptoms of chronic graft-versus-host disease. *Biology of Blood and Marrow Transplantation, 8* (8), 444-452.

Lee, S.J., Kim, H.T., Ho, V.T., Cutler, C., Alyea, E.P., Soiffer, R.J., & Antin, J.H. (2006). Quality of life associated with acute and chronic graft-versus-host disease. *Bone Marrow Transplantation, 38* (4), 305-310.

Lemaistre, C.F. & Loberiza Jr., F.R. (2005). What is quality in a transplant program? *Biology of Blood and Marrow Transplantation, 11* (4), 241-246.

Li, C.K., Lee, V., Shing, M.M., & Leung, T.F. (2009). Haematopoietic stem cell transplantation for thalassaemia in Chinese patients. *Hong Kong Medical Journal = Xianggang Yi Xue Za Zhi / Hong Kong Academy of Medicine, 15* (3 Suppl 3), 39-41.

Lim, P.A.C. & Tow, A.M. (2007). Recovery and regeneration after spinal cord injury: A review and summary of recent literature. *Annals of the Academy of Medicine Singapore, 36* (1), 49-57.

Lounsberry, J.J., Macrae, H., Angen, M., Hoeber, M., & Carlson, L.E. (2010). Feasibility study of a telehealth delivered, psychoeducational support group for allogeneic hematopoietic stem cell transplant patients. *Psycho-oncology, 19* (7), 777-781.

Malhotra, P., Hogan, W.J., Litzow, M.R., Elliott, M.A., Gastineau, D.A., Ansell, S.M., Dispenzieri, A., Gertz, M.A., Hayman, S.R., Inwards, D.J., Lacy, M.Q., Micallef, I.N., Porrata, L.F., & Tefferi, A. (2008). Long-term outcome of allogeneic stem cell transplantation in chronic lymphocytic leukemia: Analysis after a minimum follow-up of 5 years. *Leukemia and Lymphoma, 49* (9), 1724-1730.

Marmont, A.M. (1993). Immune ablation with stem-cell rescue: A possible cure for systemic lupus erythematosus? *Lupus, 2* (3), 151-156.

Marsh, J. (2006). Making therapeutic decisions in adults with aplastic anemia. *Hematology/the Education Program of the American Society of Hematology. American Society of Hematology Education Program*, 78-85.

Martinez, H.R., Gonzalez-Garza, M.T., Moreno-Cuevas, J.E., Caro, E., Gutierrez-Jimenez, E., & Segura, J.J. (2009). Stem-cell transplantation into the frontal motor cortex in amyotrophic lateral sclerosis patients. *Cytotherapy, 11* (1), 26-34.

Maschan, A.A., Skorobogatova, E.V., Kravchenko, E.G., Samochatova, E.V., Balashov, D.N., Trakhtman, P.E., Shipitsina, I.P., Pashanov, E.D., Blagonravova, O.L., Dontsenko, A.P., & Rumyantsev, A.G. (2002). Results of transplantation of hematopoetic stem cells in children with Fanconi anemia. *Gematologiya i Transfusiologiya, 47* (6), 3-6.

Mastropietro, A.P., Oliveira-Cardoso, E.A., Simões, B.P., Voltarelli, J.C., & Santos, M.A. (2010). Relationship between income, work and quality of life of patients submitted to bone marrow transplantation. *Revista Brasileira de Hematologia e Hemoterapia, 32* (2), 102-107.

McGlave, P. (1998). Unrelated donor transplant therapy for chronic myelogenous leukemia. *Hematology/oncology clinics of North America, 12* (1), 93-105.

Mengarelli, A., Iori, A.P., Romano, A., Cerretti, R., Cerilli, L., De Propris, M.S., Fenu, S., Moleti, M.L., De Felice, L., Girelli, G. & Arcese, W. (2003). One-year cyclosporine prophylaxis reduces the risk of developing extensive chronic graft-versus-host disease after allogeneic peripheral blood stem cell transplantation. *Haematologica, 88* (3), 315-323.

Messina, C., Faraci, M., De Fazio, V., Dini, G., Calò, M.P., & Calore, E. (2008). Prevention and treatment of acute GvHD. *Bone Marrow Transplantation, 41* (SUPPL. 2), S65-S70.

Messner, H.A., Curtis, J.E., Lipton, J.L., Meharchand, J.M., Minden, M.D., & Panzarella, A. (1999). Three decades of allogeneic bone marrow transplants at the Princess Margaret Hospital. *Clinical Transplants*, 289-294.

Miller, J.P., Perry, E.H., Price, T.H., Bolan Jr., C.D., Karanes, C., Boyd, T.M., Chitphakdithai, P., & King, R.J. (2008). Recovery and safety profiles of marrow and pbsc donors: experience of the national marrow donor program. *Biology of Blood and Marrow Transplantation, 14* (9 SUPPL.), 29-36.

Miller, S., Sharda, S., Rodrigue, J., & Mehta, P. (2002). Thalidomide in chronic graft-versus-host disease after stem cell transplantation: Effects on quality of life. *International Journal of Hematology, 76* (4), 365-369.

Misiak, K., Szymańska-Pomorska, G., Stawicka, M., & Wojewoda, B. (2007). Intensification of somatic symptoms after bone marrow transplant in adults as a factor influencing the subjective aspect in the elevation of health and life quality by patients. *Onkologia Polska, 10* (4), 199-202.

Moore, C.W. & Rauch, P.K. (2006). Addressing parenting concerns of bone marrow transplant patients: Opening (and closing) Pandora's box. *Bone Marrow Transplantation, 38* (12), 775-782.

Muñoz, A., Díaz-Heredia, C., Badell, I., Bureo, E., Gómez, P., Martínez, A., Verdeguer, A., Pérez-Hurtado, J.M., Fernández-Delgado, R., González-Vicent, M., & Maldonado, M.S. (2009). Allogeneic stem cell transplantation for myelodysplastic syndromes in children: A Report from the Spanish working party for blood and marrow transplantation in children (GETMON). *Pediatric Hematology and Oncology, 26* (5), 345-355.

Nagao, T. (1993). Workshop for bone marrow transplant coordinator: bone marrow transplant for pediatric patients. *[Kango] Japanese Journal of Nursing, 45* (13), 125-137.

Ness, K.K., Bhatia, S., Baker, K.S., Francisco, L., Carter, A., Forman, S.J., Robison, L.L., Rosenthal, J., & Gurney, J.G. (2005). Performance limitations and participation restrictions among childhood cancer survivors treated with hematopoietic stem cell transplantation: The bone marrow transplant survivor study. *Archives of Pediatrics and Adolescent Medicine, 159* (8), 706-713.

Nuss, S.L. & Wilson, M.E. (2007). Health-related quality of life following hematopoietic stem cell transplant during childhood. *Journal of Pediatric Oncology Nursing, 24* (2), 106-115.

Olbrisch, M.E., Benedict, S.M., Ashe, K., & Levenson, J.L. (2002). Psychological assessment and care of organ transplant patients. *Journal of Consulting and Clinical Psychology, 70* (3), 771-783.

Ortega, J.J. & Olive, T. (1998). Haematopoietic progenitor cell transplant in acute leukaemias in children: Indications, results and controversies. *Bone Marrow Transplantation, 21* (SUPPL. 2), S11-S16.

Patzer, L., Kentouche, K., Ringelmann, F., & Misselwitz, J. (2003). Renal function following hematological stem cell transplantation in childhood. *Pediatric Nephrology, 18* (7), 623-635.

Phipps, S., Dunavant, M., Garvie, P.A., Lensing, S., & Rai, S.N. (2002). Acute health-related quality of life in children undergoing stem cell transplant: I. Descriptive outcomes. *Bone Marrow Transplantation, 29* (5), 425-434.

Phipps, S., Dunavant, M., Lensing, S., & Rai, S.N. (2002). Acute health-related quality of life in children undergoing stem cell transplant: II. Medical and demographic determinants. *Bone Marrow Transplantation, 29* (5), 435-442.

Pidala, J., Anasetti, C., & Jim, H. (2010). Health-related quality of life following haematopoietic cell transplantation: Patient education, evaluation and intervention. *British Journal Of Haematology, 148* (3), 373-385.

Prasad, V.K. & Kurtzberg, J. (2010). Transplant outcomes in mucopolysaccharidoses. *Seminars in Hematology, 47* (1), 59-69.

Prasad, V.K. & Kurtzberg, J. (2008). Emerging trends in transplantation of inherited metabolic diseases. *Bone Marrow Transplantation, 41* (2), 99-108.

Ramsay, N.K., Davies, S., Wagner, J., Mcgough, E., & Mcglave, P.B. (1996). Bone marrow transplantation. New strategies for treating malignant disease. *Minnesota Medicine, 79* (4), 23-28.

Resnick, I.B., Shapira, M.Y., & Slavin, S. (2005). Nonmyeloablative stem cell transplantation and cell therapy for malignant and non-malignant diseases. *Transplant Immunology, 14* (3-4 SPEC. ISS.), 207-219.

Rodwell, R. (1996). Cord blood banking: New frontiers in stem cell therapy. *Australian Journal of Medical Science, 17* (4), 164.

Rovelli, A.M. & Steward, C.G. (2005). Hematopoietic cell transplantation activity in Europe for inherited metabolic diseases: Open issues and future directions. Bone marrow transplantation, 35(SUPPL. 1), S23-S26.

Russell, J.A., Larratt, L., Brown, C., Turner, A.R., Chaudhry, A., Booth, K., Woodman, R.C., Wolff, J., Valentine, K., Stewart, D., Ruether, J.D., Ruether, B.A., Klassen, J., Jones, A.R., Gyonyor, E., Egeler, M., Dunsmore, J., Desai, S., Coppes, M.J., Bowen, T., Anderson, R., & Poon, M.-. (1999). Allogeneic blood stem cell and bone marrow transplantation for acute myelogenous leukemia and myelodysplasia: Influence of stem cell source on outcome. *Bone Marrow Transplantation, 24* (11), 1177-1183.

Russell, J.A., Turner, A.R., Larratt, L., Chaudhry, A., Morris, D., Brown, C., Quinlan, D., & Stewart, D. (2007). Adult recipients of matched related donor blood cell transplants given myeloablative regimens including pretransplant antithymocyte globulin have lower mortality related to graft-versus-host disease: A matched pair analysis. *Biology of Blood and Marrow Transplantation, 13* (3), 299-306.

Schmitz, N., Beksac, M., Bacigalupo, A., Ruutu, T., Nagler, A., Gluckman, E., Russell, N., Apperley, J., Szer, J., Bradstock, K., Buzyn, A., Schlegelberger, B., Matcham, J., & Gratwohl, A. (2005). Filgrastim-mobilized peripheral blood progenitor cells versus bone marrow transplantation for treating leukemia: 3-year results from the EBMT randomized trial. *Haematologica, 90* (5), 643-648.

Schulmeister, L., Quiett, K., & Mayer, K. (2005). Quality of life, quality of care, and patient satisfaction: Perceptions of patients undergoing outpatient autologous stem cell transplantation. *Oncology Nursing Forum, 32* (1), 57-67.

Schwartz, R.N. & Vozniak, M. (2008). Current and emerging treatments for multiple myeloma. *Journal of Managed Care Pharmacy, 14* (7 SUPPL.), S12-S18.

Sherman, A.C., Simonton, S., Latif, U., Nieder, M.L., Adams, R.H., & Mehta, P. (2004). Psychosocial supportive care for children receiving stem cell transplantation: Practice patterns across centers. *Bone Marrow Transplantation, 34* (2), 169-174.

Sherman, R.S., Cooke, E., & Grant, M. (2005). Dialogue among survivors of hematopoietic cell transplantation: Support-group themes. *Journal of Psychosocial Oncology, 23* (1), 1-24.

Silani, V. & Cova, L. (2008). Stem cell transplantation in multiple sclerosis: Safety and ethics. *Journal of the Neurological Sciences, 265* (1-2), 116-121.

Silverman, L.R. (2004). DNA methyltransferase inhibitors in myelodysplastic syndrome. *Best Practice and Research: Clinical Haematology, 17* (4 SPEC.ISS.), 585-594.

Sinha, R. & Lonial, S. (2006). Novel treatment approaches for patients with relapsed and refractory multiple myeloma. *Current Treatment Options in Oncology, 7* (3), 246-257.

Sirohi, B. & Powles, R. (2001). High-dose therapy in patients with multiple myeloma. *Oncology Spectrums, 2* (2), 86-95.

Smith, E.P. & Nademanee, A. (1995). Bone marrow transplantation: the City of Hope experience. *Clinical Transplants*, 291-310.

Snowden, J.A., Martin-Rendon, E. & Watt, S.M. (2009). Clinical stem cell therapies for severe autoimmune diseases. *Transfusion Medicine, 19* (5), 223-234.

Souillet, G. (1998). Indications and results of progenitor cell transplant in congenital haemopathies (except Fanconi anaemia). *Bone Marrow Transplantation, 21* (SUPPL. 2), S28-S33.

Spurr, E.E., Wiggins, N.E., Marsden, K.A., Lowenthal, R.M. & Ragg, S.J. (2002). Cryopreserved human haematopoietic stem cells retain engraftment potential after extended (5-14 years) cryostorage. *Cryobiology, 44* (3), 210-217.

Spyridonidis, A., Schmidt, M., Bernhardt, W., Papadimitriou, A., Azemar, M., Wels, W., Groner, B., & Henschler, R. (1998). Purging of mammary carcinoma cells during ex vivo culture of CD34+ hematopoietic progenitor cells with recombinant immunotoxins. *Blood, 91* (5), 1820-1827.

Srinivasan, S. & Schiffer, C.A., (2008). Current treatment options and strategies for myelodysplastic syndromes. *Expert Opinion on Pharmacotherapy, 9* (10), 1667-1678.

Stephens, J.M., Gramegna, P., Laskin, B., Botteman, M.F., & Pashos, C.L. (2005). Chronic lymphocytic leukemia: Economic burden and quality of life: Literature review. *American Journal of Therapeutics, 12* (5), 460-466.

Tallman, B., Shaw, K., Schultz, J., & Altmaier, E. (2010). well-being and posttraumatic growth in unrelated donor marrow transplant survivors: A nine-year longitudinal study. *Rehabilitation Psychology, 55* (2), 204-210.

Tang, J.L., Yao, M., Lu, M.Y., Ko, B.S., Lin, D.T., Lin, K.H., & Chen, Y.C. (2009). Long-term outcome of allogeneic human leukocyte antigen-matched sibling-donor peripheral blood stem cell transplantation in leukaemia patients. *Hong Kong Medical Journal = Xianggang Yi Xue Za Zhi / Hong Kong Academy Of Medicine, 15* (3 Suppl 3), 31-34.

Tierney, D.K., Facione, N., Padilla, G., & Dodd, M., (2007). Response shift: A theoretical exploration of quality of life following hematopoietic cell transplantation. *Cancer Nursing, 30* (2), 125-138.

Tirindelli, M.C., Flammia, G., Sergi, F., Cerretti, R., Cudillo, L., Picardi, A., Postorino, M., Annibali, O., Greco, R., Avvisati, G., & Arcese, W. (2009). Fibrin glue for refractory hemorrhagic cystitis after unrelated marrow, cord blood, and haploidentical hematopoietic stem cell transplantation. *Transfusion, 49* (1), 170-175.

Van Der Laarse, A., Umar, S., Steendijk, P., Ypey, D.L., Atsma, D.E., Van Der Wall, E.E., & Schalij, M.J. (2010). Novel approaches to treat experimental pulmonary arterial hypertension: A review. *Journal of Biomedicine and Biotechnology*, 2010.

Van Hennik, P.B., Breems, D.A., Withagen, C.M., Slaper, I.C.M., & Plogmacher, R.E. (1997). Graft-failure can be predicted by testing the ability of stem cells to produce progenitors in long-term stroma-supported cultures. *Experimental Hematology, 25* (8), 742.

Verma, S., Younus, J., Haynes, A.E., Stys-Norman, D., & Blackstein, M. (2008). Dose-intensive chemotherapy with growth factor or autologous bone marrow or stem-cell transplant support in first-line treatment of advanced or metastatic adult soft tissue sarcoma: A clinical practice guideline. *Current Oncology, 15* (2), 31-35.

Vogelsang, G.B., & Higman, M.A. (2004). Chronic graft versus host disease. *British Journal of Haematology, 125* (4), 435-454.

Voltarelli, J.C., Stracieri, A.B.P.L., Oliveira, M.C.B., Godoi, D.F., Moraes, D.A., Pieroni, F., Malmegrim, K.C.R., Coutinho, M.A., & Simões, B.P. (2005). Hematopoietic stem cell transplantation for rheumatic diseases. Part 1: International experience. *Revista Brasileira de Reumatologia, 45* (4), 229-241.

Weisdorf, D., Carter, S., Confer, D., Ferrara, J., & Horowitz, M. (2007). Blood and marrow transplant clinical trials network (bmt ctn): Addressing unanswered questions. *Biology of Blood and Marrow Transplantation, 13* (3), 257-262.

Wingard, J.R., Moreb, J.S., & Gaa, R.I. (1999). High-dose chemotherapy with autologous stem cell rescue as a treatment modality for breast cancer. *Breast Journal, 5* (5), 308-318.

Wong, R., Giralt, S.A., Martin, T., Couriel, D.R., Anagnostopoulos, A., Hosing, C., Andersson, B.S., Cano, P., Shahjahan, M., Ippoliti, C., Estey, E.H., Mcmannis, J., Gajewski, J.L., Champlin, R.E., & De Lima, M., (2003). Reduced-intensity conditioning for unrelated donor hematopoietic stem cell transplantation as treatment for myeloid malignancies in patients older than 55 years. *Blood, 102* (8), 3052-3059.

Worel, N., Keil, F., Kalhs, P., Biener, D., Mitterbauer, M., Rabitsch, W., Hoecker, P., Lechner, K., & Greinix, H. (2000). Long term outcome of patients who are alive and in complete remission two years after allogeneic stem cell transplantation. *Blood, 96* (11 PART I).

Zantomio, D., Grigg, A.P., Macgregor, L., Panek-Hudson, Y., Szer, J., & Ayton, R. (2006). Female genital tract graft-versus-host disease: Incidence, risk factors and recommendations for management. *Bone Marrow Transplantation, 38* (8), 567-572.

www.ingramcontent.com/pod-product-compliance
Lightning Source LLC
Chambersburg PA
CBHW080230200526
45165CB00026B/3446